Quick
Workouts
Fitness on the Go

FITNESS, HEALTH & NUTRITION

Quick
Workouts

Fitness on the Go

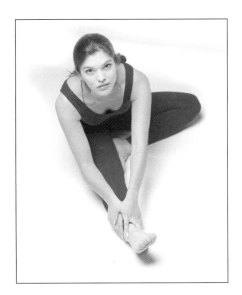

TIME®
LIFE

by the Editors of Time-Life Books

CONSULTANTS FOR THIS BOOK

William D. McArdle, Ph.D., is a professor in the Department of Health and Physical Education at Queens College of the City University of New York. Dr. McArdle is a Fellow of the American College of Sports Medicine. He is Consulting Exercise Physiologist to Weight Watchers International, Inc., and *Weight Watchers Magazine*. Among his books are *Exercise Physiology: Energy, Nutrition and Human Performance, Getting in Shape* and *Nutrition, Weight Control, and Exercise.*

William B. Zuti, Ph.D., is the Director of the Pepsico Fitness Center at Pepsico, Inc., Purchase, N.Y. he is fellow and Treasurer of the American College of Sports Medicine; a Fellow of the Association for Fitness in Business; and a member of the Research Council of the American Alliance of Health, Physical Education and Dance. He is the author and co-author of many books including *Administration of Physical Fitness Programs, Health* and *The Official YMCA Fitness Program.*

Ann Grandjean M.S., is Associate Director of the Swanson Center for Nutrition, Omaha, Neb.; chief nutrition consultant to the U.S. Olympic committee; and an instructor in the Sports Medicine Program, Orthopedic Surgery Department, University of Nebraska Medical Center.

Myron Winick, M.D., is the R.R. Williams Professor of Nutrition, Professor of Pediatrics, Director of the Institute of Human Nutrition, and Director of the Center for Nutrition, Genetics and Human Development at Columbia University College of Physicians and Surgeons. He has served on the Food and Nutrition Board of the National Academy of Sciences and is the author of many books, including *Your Personalized Health Profile.*

The following consultants helped design the exercise sequences in this book:

Nancy Klitsner, who holds a master's degree in applied physiology, is an exercise physiologist in private practice in New York City. She consults with corporations and schools on developing fitness programs and conducts a certification-training program for exercise instructors. Ms. Klitsner is co-owner of Klitsner/Mello Associates, a corporate stress management business

Jessica Wolf has been a certified Alexander teacher from the American Center for the Alexander Technique in New York City since 1977. She is also a certified Movement Analyst from the Laban Institute. In addition to maintaining a private practice, she teaches at colleges throughout the United States, including Hunter College in New York.

This edition published in 2004
by the Caxton Publishing Group
20 Bloomsbury Street, London WC1B 3JH

Under license from Time-Life Books BV.

Cover Design: Open Door Limited, Rutland UK

Title: Quick Workouts

ISBN: 1 84447 160 8

This book is not intended as a substitute for the advice of a physician. Readers who have or suspect they have specific medical problems, especially those involving muscles and joints, should consult a physician before beginning any programme of strenuous physical exercise.

CONTENTS

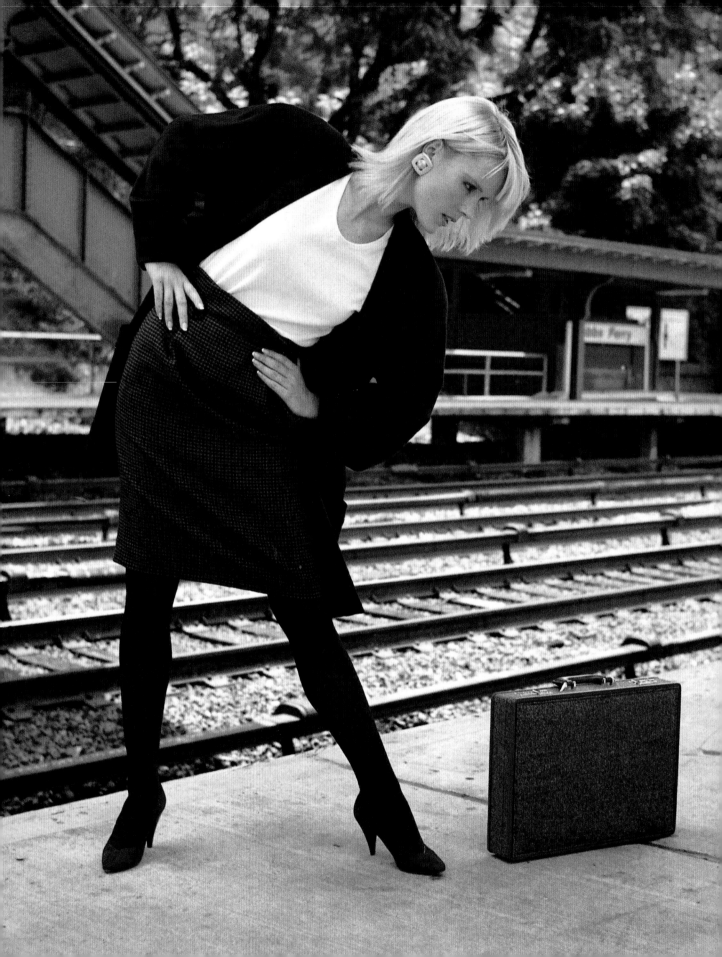

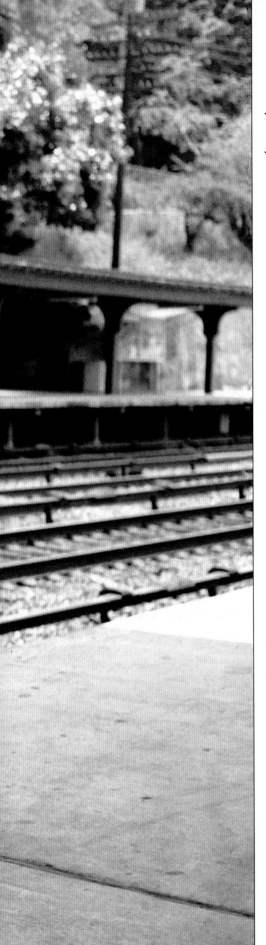

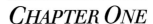
Fitness Any Time, Anywhere

*Preserving the benefits
of exercise with workouts that
are efficient, comprehensive —
and brief*

Lack of time is the most common explanation that people offer for giving up an exercise programme. But few people realize that, even if they do not have time for intensive workouts, it is possible to stay fit with an abbreviated exercise routine. Once you have achieved a moderate level of fitness, you can maintain it despite a busy schedule. Even if you spend long hours working in an office or caring for children at home, or if your working week is often interrupted by business travel, there are exercises that you can do virtually anywhere to keep yourself in shape. Those who let their training lapse may face the challenge of re-establishing the benefits they have lost, which demands much more time and energy than merely maintaining fitness.

What is a quick workout?
First and foremost, a quick workout is an efficient exercise routine that provides the maximum fitness benefits in a brief time. The key to its effectiveness is the intensity of each exercise — that is, how hard you exert yourself. By increasing the intensity, you can decrease the

7

The Fitness Fall-Off Rate

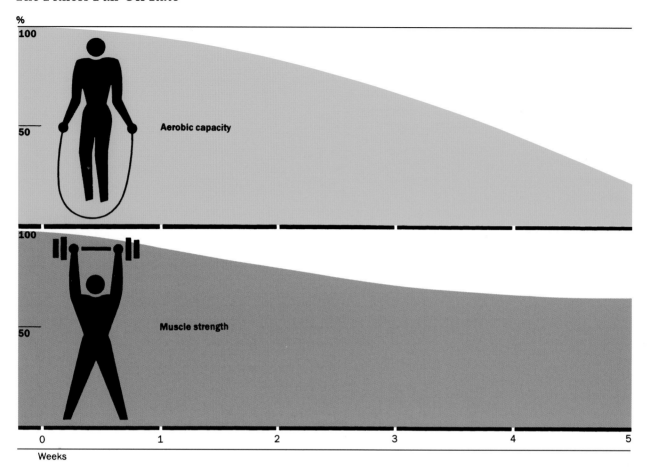

%

Aerobic capacity

Muscle strength

Weeks

Two chief elements of fitness — aerobic capacity and muscle strength — will decline if exercise stops. As the chart above shows, the drop in aerobic capacity averages about 10 to 15 per cent after two weeks without exercise; nearly 80 per cent of fitness improvements are lost after five weeks, according to several studies. Muscle strength may last longer than aerobic capacity: subjects in one study had only a 35 per cent drop in their strength gains after five weeks without exercise.

amount of time you devote to an exercise — whether it be a set of push-ups or an aerobics routine — and thus reap the benefits more rapidly. Although quick workouts are most useful for those times when your usual exercise schedule is disrupted — when travelling, for example, or putting in extra hours at work — you can perform a quick workout if you have only limited time to devote to exercise. The quick workouts shown in this book can be done in just 20 minutes, a period of time that even the busiest schedule can accommodate.

Do quick workouts provide a total fitness regimen?
A 20-minute workout does not constitute a complete fitness programme. So, for maximum results, each workout should be devoted either to aerobic or strength exercises, but not both. And each type of exercise should be accompanied by stretches for flexibility, an easy cardiovascular warm-up and a cool-down.

Most exercise experts believe that while strength, flexibility and aerobic training are all crucial for total fitness, aerobic exercise is the most important. Aerobic exercise includes such vigorous endurance activities as running, walking, cycling and swimming, which work large muscle groups and condition your cardiovascular system, producing physiological changes that are referred to collectively as a training effect. If your time is severely restricted, you should devote all or most of your workouts to aerobic exercise. But whenever possible, you should arrange a schedule that allows you to switch between aerobics and strength exercises on alternate days, or to fit two quick workouts — one aerobic, the other for strength — into a 40-minute exercise session three times a week.

Can you really get an effective aerobic workout in only 20 minutes?

The effectiveness of a workout depends on how fit you already are. If you are out of shape, you should exercise aerobically for 30 minutes at least three times a week to build up your fitness level. Such a workout begins with a five-minute warm-up and concludes with five minutes of cool-down and stretching. According to recent findings by exercise physiologists, working out less than this produces little or no training effect in unconditioned individuals.

Once you have achieved an acceptable level of aerobic fitness, which generally takes two to six months for someone who is healthy but has not exercised consistently for several years, you can maintain it with less exercise. In one study, aerobically fit subjects were able to stay in shape by exercising every third day. In another study, exercising just twice a week was sufficient to maintain aerobic capacity in a group of fit subjects. In that same study, exercising even once a week was found to help slow the decline of fitness, although a weekly workout was insufficient to maintain fitness at optimal levels. Other research shows that endurance training at low intensity less frequently than twice a week and for less than 10 minutes per session is not adequate for fitness maintenance.

If you are out of shape, will quick workouts offer any benefit?

For people who exercise rarely or not at all, short but frequent bouts of aerobic exertion can improve fitness to some extent. In one study, for example, sedentary subjects were able to increase their aerobic capacity by approximately 15 per cent in three months by running on the spot for just 10 minutes a day.

Nevertheless, it requires more effort to get into shape than it does to maintain fitness once you have achieved it. Most exercise experts advise people who are out of shape to undertake an exercise programme slowly but steadily. The programme should become increasingly demanding over a period of months, aiming to reach your optimal level of cardiovascular conditioning.

Brief aerobic workouts must be performed at a relatively high level of intensity (measured in terms of heart rate) to be beneficial. Unfit individuals should not start exercising at such levels. Studies show that engaging abruptly or sporadically in any vigorous activity — shovelling snow, for example — may increase the risk of heart attack in

How Much is Enough?

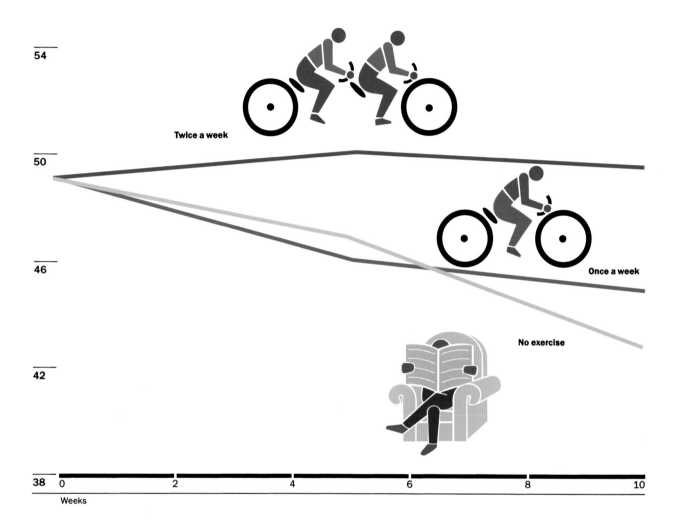

VO$_2$Max

58

54

50

46

42

38   0   2   4   6   8   10

Weeks

Twice a week

Once a week

No exercise

It takes less time per week to maintain fitness than to build it. The graph above shows the results of a study of subjects who performed a 10-week maintenance programme after they had trained three times a week to build aerobic fitness. During their training, the subjects' average VO$_2$max had increased from a low point of 38 to nearly 50. When the subjects cut back their training, those who worked out twice a week were able to maintain their fitness gains. Subjects who cut back to once a week showed a noticeable decline in aerobic capacity, but were still in better shape than those who stopped exercising.

sedentary people, particularly those with unidentified coronary problems. Being out of shape also increases the likelihood of muscle or joint injury during an intense workout. Therefore, quick workouts are best suited to maintaining fitness in those who are already fit.

If you stop exercising, how quickly will you lose aerobic fitness?

The benefits acquired over months or years do not vanish overnight when an exercise programme is interrupted, but the effects of aerobic conditioning are definitely reversible. A number of studies have found that VO$_2$max, a measure of aerobic fitness that reflects the maximum volume of oxygen the body can take in and use per minute of intense exercise, drops by up to 10 to 15 per cent after two weeks without any aerobic exercise at all. After four to 12 weeks of not exercising — which physiologists refer to as detraining — participants in one study experienced a 50 per cent drop in their VO_2max.

Scientists believe that this loss of cardiovascular conditioning varies from person to person. The speed at which your fitness drops off during a slack period also depends on how well trained you were when you gave up exercising: if two people stop exercising for the same amount of time, the person who was fit for only a few days or weeks will drop to a lower level of fitness, as measured in VO_2max, than someone who had been fit for a year or more. Still, researchers note that even a highly trained athlete who stops working out will, over the course of several months, lose all the fitness gains that he or she had achieved through training.

How long does it take to regain aerobic fitness?
It takes about as long to retrain your cardiovascular system as it takes to become aerobically fit in the first place. There is apparently no transfer of fitness benefits from one training period to the next if a significant period of detraining has intervened. A study of students who had increased their aerobic capacity during seven weeks of training, for example, showed that seven additional weeks without exercise decreased their aerobic capacity to within 3 per cent of their pre-training levels. Afterwards, it took them another seven weeks to regain the fitness level they had lost. Clearly, it is much more efficient to use quick workouts to maintain fitness than to stop exercising until detraining has become almost complete.

Are strength and flexibility lost as easily as aerobic fitness?
Few studies have been done on strength retention. However, the research that has been done suggests that it takes longer to lose strength and flexibility than it does to lose aerobic capacity: one study found that, without strength-building exercise, muscular power undergoes a slow, steady decline resulting in a 35 per cent loss in five weeks.

Similarly, maintaining muscular strength is less time consuming than maintaining aerobic fitness. In fact, in an experiment using isometric exercises, which are described below, participants needed to exercise just once every other week to maintain the gains they had attained during a daily training regimen.

The data on flexibility are scant, but many exercise scientists believe that muscles deprived of exercise grow shorter. And the longer you neglect your muscles, the shorter and less flexible they become.

What is the quickest way to build strength?
Isometric, or static, exercises, in which you contract muscles against a fixed resistance, such as a wall, take only a few seconds to perform. Moreover, they require no equipment and are inconspicuous enough to

be done any time, anywhere. In addition, an isometric workout can substantially boost your muscle strength. In one particular study, subjects using isometrics were able to increase the power of a hand muscle by an average of 51 per cent, compared to a 19 per cent gain among subjects doing another type of strengthening exercise. The gains from isometrics are also much easier to maintain than aerobic capacity: most experts agree that working out isometrically once a week is enough for maintenance.

Isometric exercise is not without its drawbacks, however. Most important, muscular development achieved by isometrics occurs only at the specific angle within a joint's range of motion at which force is applied *(see illustration, page 14)*. Therefore, to gain strength uniformly, even within the same muscle group, you must perform isometric contractions at four or five angles throughout the joint's range of motion. Although each contraction takes only a few seconds, repeating it in a number of positions obviously prolongs your workout. In addition, researchers have found that blood pressure tends to shoot up during and just after an isometric contraction. Doctors therefore warn heart patients and anyone with high blood pressure to avoid isometrics, as well as other strenuous strengthening exercises such as weight lifting.

Do quick workouts effectively yield long-term health benefits?
Research suggests that any kind of exercise, even in small doses, improves overall health and lengthens life expectancy. One of the most comprehensive longevity studies ever undertaken — a 20-year survey of nearly 17,000 Harvard graduates by Dr. Ralph S. Paffenbarger Jr. and his associates — revealed that even a moderate amount of physical activity, particularly when it has an aerobic component, made a difference. In his study, men who expended 500 to 1,000 calories a week — roughly the equivalent of walking eight to 16 kilometres a week, or about 20 minutes a day — had a 22 per cent lower risk of death than those who got no exercise at all (a group the researchers used as a benchmark for assigning a 100 per cent risk of death).

Is there a best time of day to exercise?
Almost any time is fine, as long as it fits into your schedule. However, you should not exercise vigorously just after a meal, when your blood is at work absorbing nutrients from your food and therefore not as readily available to flow to your muscles. Nor should you perform aerobic exercise just before going to bed, as such exercise stimulates the release of adrenaline, a hormone that may keep you awake.

Some evidence does suggest that people who exercise in the morning tend to stay with their exercise routines more consistently than those who work out at other times of day. And many corporate fitness-programme directors have found that the morning is virtually the only time a busy person can fit exercise into his or her schedule, especially if the working day extends into the evening.

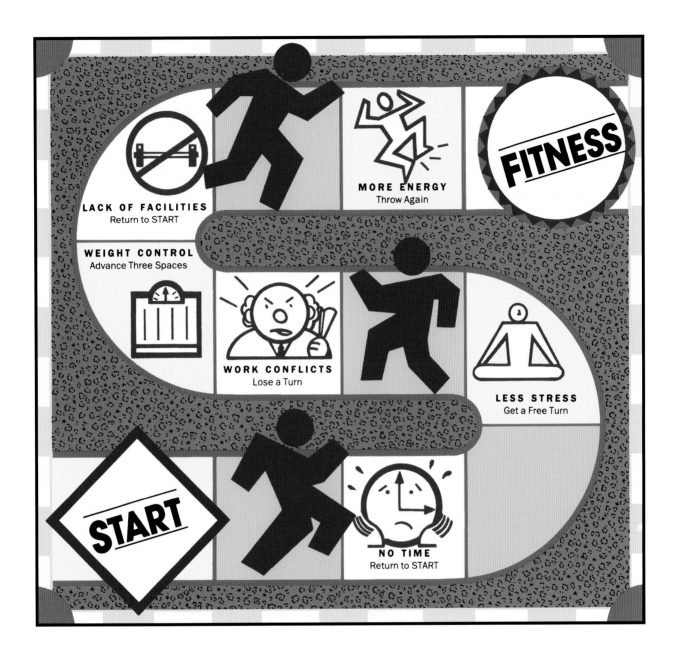

The Game of Fitness

Between 40 and 50 per cent of people who enrol in supervised exercise programmes drop out in the first six to 12 months. The biggest obstacle to sticking to an exercise programme is insufficient time. In one survey, nearly half the drop-outs gave lack of time as their reason for stopping. In another survey that polled people who did not exercise, 40 per cent said they would do so if they had more time.

Lack of facilities and work conflicts are other obstacles that people commonly cite. Further evidence that convenience is a key factor in staying with a programme comes from a Canadian study of 13,500 households. The researchers found that the most popular forms of exercise are walking, cycling, swimming, jogging, gardening and exercises that can be done at home. All of these activities require little or no equipment and fit easily into almost any schedule.

Another incentive for adhering to an exercise programme is to remember the benefits that exercise provides. In the Canadian study, respondents said exercise makes you more energetic, reduces stress and helps control weight.

Isometrics: The Quickest Workout of All?

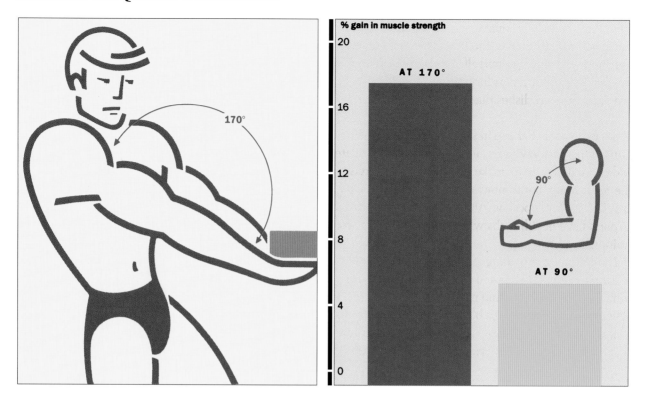

% gain in muscle strength

AT 170°

90°

AT 90°

Isometric exercises are quick: you can strengthen and tone a muscle by contracting it against a stationary object — such as a shelf or wall — for just six seconds. But there are limitations to isometrics. In one study, subjects performed an isometric contraction with their arms at a 170-degree angle *(above)*. After six weeks, their muscle strength had increased by 18 per cent, but only when measured with the arm at the same 170-degree angle. When arm strength was measured with the elbow at 90 degrees, the gain was only 5 per cent *(above, right)*. To use isometrics effectively, see pages 74-75.

If you do not have time for even a quick workout, can other day-to-day activities help maintain fitness?

Any vigorous physical activity will help you stay fit, whether it is part of a formal exercise programme or connected with your job or your leisure-time pursuits. Within the scope of your daily routine, there are many ways to create opportunities for exercise to develop your aerobic fitness as well as your strength and flexibility.

A primary requirement for deriving aerobic benefits is that you perform an activity at a pace that would burn 200 to 400 calories in an hour *(for examples see pages 18-19)*. You can accomplish this with activities usually considered to be exercise, such as running, but raking leaves, gardening or scrubbing a floor can be done vigorously enough to give you a workout as well.

You can also develop or maintain strength with ordinary everyday tasks. Books and other objects can be used for dynamic strength exercises, as shown in Chapter Three. Or, if you have no items available that you can lift or move around, you can perform isometric exercises anywhere or at any time by simply opposing one part of your body with another or by pressing against an immovable object.

How can you maintain a healthy diet while you are on the go?

Unfortunately, many of the dishes served in fast-food restaurants, cafés and pubs are high in fat, salt and sugar. For example, fast-food establishments typically fry fish in shortening; as a result, fish burgers may derive more than 50 per cent of their calories from fat. Fried fish also may have substantial amounts of sugar and salt added to the batter. If you have the time, the best way to ensure that a quick meal will be nutritious is to make it yourself ahead of time and take it with you. Chapter Five contains tips for ordering food in restaurants as well as advice on preparing healthy dishes that are easy to make and portable.

What can you do to keep in shape when you travel?
During the past few years, many businesses that cater for travellers have added facilities that make it easier to exercise while you are on the road. Many hotels now either offer exercise rooms and equipment or are affiliated with local health clubs that hotel guests are free to use. Some airports have health clubs where it is possible to work out while you are waiting for a flight.

In addition to providing guidebooks that include information on where to exercise, some hotels and motels will advise runners about safe routes; some even provide jogging maps with distances marked. You can inquire at your hotel about hiring a bicycle or cross-country skis, or you can consult a local telephone directory. You can also use your hotel or motel room as a personal gym for quick workouts. The exercises in Chapter Two are designed for this purpose.

How much equipment do you need?
Most of the quick workouts described in this volume require little or no equipment. As a rule, you will need a pair of running or aerobic shoes, a T-shirt, shorts, a towel and, for some of the exercises, a table, chair and some light weights.

How can you ensure that you will keep to an exercise programme?
The best way to stay motivated is to set aside time for exercise within an existing framework of activity. A recent Gallup poll showed that people who find the time to exercise regularly tend to squeeze it into their schedules, rather than altering their routines by getting up earlier or otherwise changing their lives.

More advice on how to fit exercise into your daily life is offered on page 19. To assess your current activity level and design a programme that meets your needs and your schedule, turn to the next page.

How to Design Your Own Programme

itting exercise and healthy eating into a busy schedule is never easy. But it is not impossible. If your lifestyle, your job and frequent travel have interfered with your exercise programme, the first step towards staying in shape is to assess your daily routines.

The questions on these two pages not only indicate the circumstances that may sidetrack you, but also suggest ways to turn them into opportunities. Before long, you will be able to see other ways of getting around many apparent obstacles to maintaining your fitness routine.

How busy are you?

1 Do you sit all day at your job?

To stay healthy, you need to stay active, day in and day out. The more sedentary your job, the more you may need a fitness programme that can help counteract the harmful effects of sitting for hours on end. Studies of university graduates, dockers and civil servants conducted over periods of up to 20 years have shown that those men who were more active, either at work or during their leisure time, had lower rates of heart disease and certain types of cancer than their less active counterparts. These same studies have also shown that even activities that require only moderate exertion, such as gardening, can dramatically reduce the risk of heart disease when they are performed regularly. If you get through most working days without much physical exertion, quick workouts can compensate for your lack of on-the-job exercise.

If you can incorporate exercise into your normal routine, you will have a better chance of following through on your programme than if you feel compelled to get up earlier or cut short another activity. The tips on page 19 explain how you can fit exercise into your day.

2 How do you get to work?

If you commute by car, train or bus, you may be overlooking an opportunity to work exercise into your schedule. Exercising while you commute is one of the simplest ways of exerting yourself without devoting much extra time to a physical fitness programme. If possible, ride a bike, walk or run instead of driving a car or taking public transport. Of course, that may not be practical if you live far from work or in a heavily urbanized area. But even small increases in activities such as walking and climbing stairs can produce significant health benefits over time. In the study of university graduates mentioned above, increasing the number of stairs climbed weekly was associated with increased longevity. A minor shift in your routine, such as parking your car several blocks from the office and briskly walking for 10 to 20 minutes daily, can also add up to a major fitness advantage.

3 Do you travel frequently on business?

Since a well-established routine is the key to a consistent, long-term exercise programme, a schedule that is often interrupted by business travel can play havoc with your fitness regimen. However, adhering to a fitness programme away from home is possible with a minimum of effort and planning. Before you travel, pack exercise clothing and shoes appropriate for the 20-minute workout shown in Chapter Two, which you can perform in your hotel room.

Always exercise on the first morning after you arrive at your destination. This can help you acclimatize to a new time zone and may establish an early morning exercise routine you can follow while you are on the road. Many fitness experts recommend exercising first thing in the morning when you are travelling to take advantage of the only free time most business travellers have.

4   How often do you dine at restaurants or eat fast food?

People who travel frequently tend to eat out a great deal, and the meals they eat may be higher in fat than the ones they eat at home. Diets high in fat are also usually high in calories and may be related to a variety of diseases, including heart disease, obesity and some kinds of cancer.

Although it is impractical to take food with you when you travel, many airlines will provide a special menu, if you request one in advance. As for meals during the working day, taking food with you to the office may be advisable. The recipes in Chapter Five offer a variety of nutritious, convenient meals that can readily be transported.

If you dine at a restaurant or eat fast food, ask for sauces and dressings to be served separately so that you can control the amounts. Order meat, fish and poultry grilled rather than fried, and choose skimmed milk, semi-skimmed milk or buttermilk rather than whole milk. See Chapter Five for more advice on eating a healthy diet while on the go.

5   Do you work long hours?

You can fit exercise into even the busiest and most unpredictable schedule if you know how — during lulls in your business day, while you are waiting in queues and while you are travelling between appointments.

You can develop strength, flexibility and, to some extent, aerobic capacity by exercising at your desk following the routines described in Chapter Three. If you have a succession of appointments throughout the day, walking from one place to the next, if time permits, may also produce long-term exercise benefits. The tension-releasing effects of walking may even make you feel more relaxed with business associates and clients.

If you feel that you do not have enough time for family and friends, and you try to embark on a strenuous exercise programme that places additional demands on your time anyway, exercise may do you more harm than good. In such circumstances, it may become another source of stress rather than a healthy release. The activities shown in the following three chapters will show you the way to maintain a fitness regimen without requiring you to forego other obligations and pleasures.

CYCLING	RUNNING	WALKING UPHILL
8 kilometres	3 kilometres	2.5 kilometres

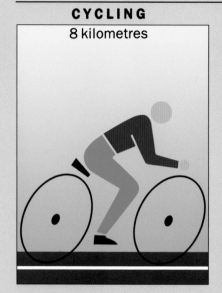 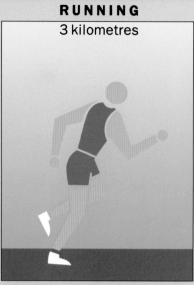 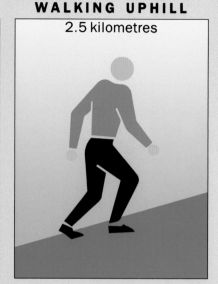

Using Intensity

There are three elements you can adjust while exercising: frequency (how often you exercise), duration (how long you perform a particular routine) and intensity (how hard you push yourself). Recent studies indicate that intensity is the most important of the three in maintaining aerobic fitness, the type of fitness most beneficial to cardiovascular health.

In one study, aerobically trained subjects were able to maintain their fitness levels when they reduced the workout frequency from six days a week to two days but still exercised at the same intensity and for the same duration. Another group of trained subjects continued to work out at the same frequency for the same duration, but lowered the intensity of their workouts by two thirds (as measured by their heart rates during exercise). After 15 weeks, those in the second group had entirely lost the aerobic capacity that

their training had produced originally. Knowing how intensely you exercise, therefore, is crucial to the success of quick workouts.

One way of measuring intensity is the amount of energy you expend in the form of kilocalories, more popularly known as calories. A kilocalorie is the heat required to raise the temperature of one gram of water by one degree Celsius. For an effective aerobic workout, exercise physiologists advise that you should exert yourself vigorously enough to burn 200 to 400 calories. To be aerobic, this exertion must be continuous and rhythmic. For some of the most common aerobic activities, the illustrations above indicate the pace you should set to accomplish this in 20 minutes. (The precise number of calories you use will vary slightly, depending on your weight. Heavier people burn more calories per minute when they exercise at the same pace as people who weigh less.)

SKIING	**SKIPPING**	**SWIMMING**
2 kilometres cross-country	60-70 jumps per minute	700-750 metres

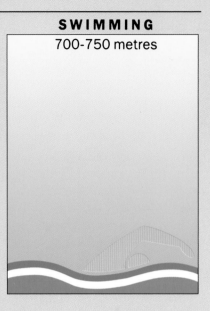

Managing Time

In survey after survey, the main reason people cite for stopping an exercise programme — or for not starting one — is lack of time. They think that exercising requires setting aside inconveniently large blocks of time that will interfere with their other activities. But most people actually do have enough time in their schedules for exercise: the key is to learn how best to manage that time. One approach is to design an exercise routine that is as convenient as possible. Several studies indicate that people whose exercise regimens require little equipment and can be done at home, at work or nearby are more likely to keep to it than those whose regimens are less convenient.

The chapters that follow contain routines that not only offer you convenience in terms of location and requiring minimal equipment, but also afford you the most fitness benefits in the least amount of time.

In addition to these quick workouts, here are a few tips for squeezing exercise into a tight schedule:

1. Walk or cycle to and from work. Or, if you have to drive or take public transport, stop a distance from work and walk briskly the rest of the way — you will burn about 50 calories per kilometre.

2. Use stairs instead of escalators or lifts. Climbing stairs requires 15 times the energy that walking on level ground does.

3. Spend your lunch hour or coffee break walking briskly or performing one of the office workouts from Chapter Three. Aerobic exercise at lunchtime can also diminish your appetite so that you eat less, an aid to those trying to lose weight.

4. Instead of sitting down while watching television, run on the spot, use an exercise bicycle, rowing machine or ski exerciser, or perform callisthenics and stretches.

Choosing an Exercise

There are four categories of exercises that you can use in a fitness programme: dynamic strength exercises, isometric exercises, stretches and aerobics. This book contains versions of all four types that are designed to be performed in special circumstances — when your schedule is tight, when you are at the office, or when you are travelling. Many of the exercises can be adapted to various situations. When you are travelling on a train, for example, you can perform some of the exercises from the office workout in Chapter Three, as well as the routine for travel shown in Chapter Four. Conversely, many of the exercises designed for travel are also well suited to an office setting.

The guide on the opposite page can help you choose exercises to fit almost any circumstance. For each type of exercise, there are seated variations, which are ideal for performing at your desk or while travelling by plane or train, as well as standing variations. Some of the standing exercises are designed to be part of a regular workout, whereas others are better suited for spare time or idle moments, such as while you are standing in a queue. A few of the strengthening and stretching routines require lying on the floor.

For the most versatile fitness programme, you should vary your routine so that you perform different types of exercise on a regular basis, as shown in the chapters that follow.

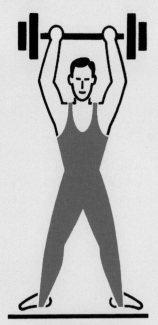

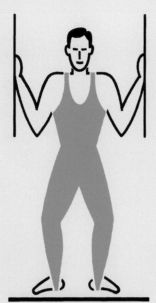

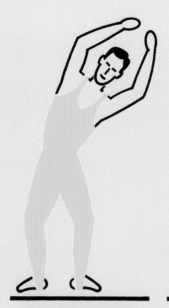

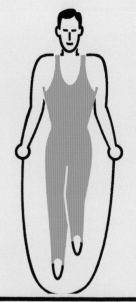

| DYNAMIC STRENGTH | ISOMETRIC EXERCISES | STRETCHING EXERCISES | AEROBIC EXERCISES |

All muscle-building exercises that involve movement are termed dynamic strength training (or isotonics). Leg lifts, sit-ups, push-ups, lifting weights and working on weight machines are in this category. These movements build strength throughout the range of motion used in the exercises.

SEATED DYNAMICS
pages 29, 50, 66-68, 70-73, 105-107

STANDING DYNAMICS
pages 43-44, 69, 114-117, 122-123

FLOOR EXERCISES
pages 30-31, 34-35, 38-42

Strength-building exercises in which the muscles remain motionless, or static, are called isometrics. During these exercises, the muscles contract against the resistance of an immovable object or other muscles. Each isometric exercise develops significant strength primarily at the position of contraction.

SEATED ISOMETRICS
pages 74-75, 98-104, 108-109

STANDING ISOMETRICS
pages 118-121

Stretches promote flexibility and lengthen a muscle by gently extending it. Stretching also relaxes muscles and can prevent or alleviate muscular soreness.

SEATED STRETCHES
pages 47, 60-63, 92-97

STANDING STRETCHES
pages 27, 45-46, 48-49, 51-53, 64-65, 112-113

FLOOR EXERCISES
pages 28, 30-33, 36-37, 45

Vigorous exercises such as running, swimming and skipping are aerobic when they continue long enough to work the body's large muscle groups and place a sustained demand on the cardiovascular system.

SEATED AEROBICS
pages 76-87

STANDING AEROBICS
pages 54-55

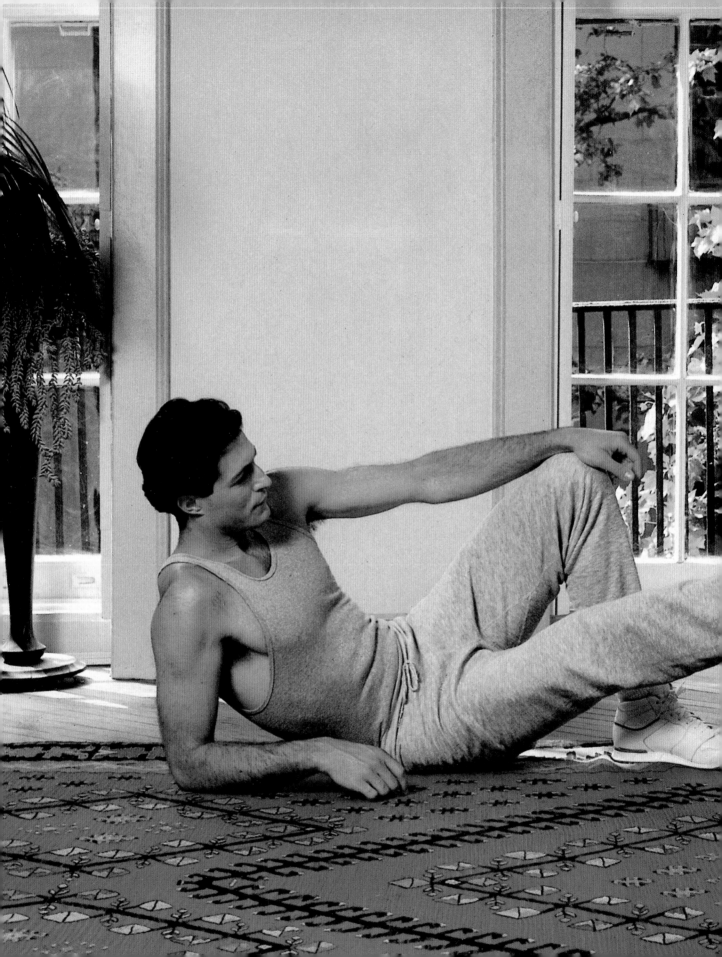

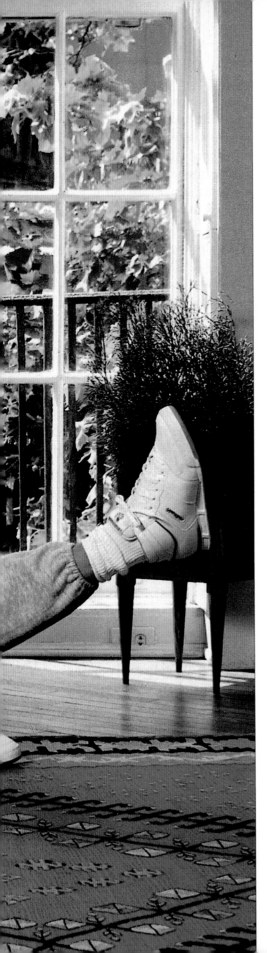

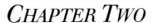
The 20-Minute Workout

A total-body regimen for strength, flexibility and endurance

The effectiveness of a fitness programme is often perceived as directly proportional to the amount of time spent exercising. But, in fact, it is possible to maintain your level of fitness with workouts that take only 20 minutes each. A thorough programme should include exercises that strengthen and tone muscles as well as aerobic routines that benefit the heart and lungs. You can perform these two types of exercises on alternate days. Or you can combine them into one longer workout that you should perform two or, better still, three days a week. And, whenever you perform strengthening or aerobic exercises, you should incorporate warm-ups, cool-downs and flexibility-enhancing movements.

The exercises shown on pages 26-53 provide a workout that lasts 20 minutes. This workout focuses on strengthening and stretching all of the body's major muscle groups. It maximizes the benefits you can derive in 20 minutes and minimizes the equipment you need. A few of the exercises require light weights, for which you can substitute commonplace items such as books. (Travellers may wish to use hollow weights that they can fill with water in their hotel rooms.) The only other equipment the exercises in this chapter call for are such readily available items as towels, tables and chairs.

The 20-minute workout includes warm-up and cool-down exercises. Many people, in an effort to save time, overlook or dispense with these two essential components, but they should not be eliminated. Warm-ups, on the one hand, are meant to loosen cold muscles gradually and increase their temperature without causing undue stress. When your muscles are more pliant, the benefits you derive from strengthening exercises increase. Once your muscles are warmed up, their range of motion expands considerably, and you can perform the exercises more effectively.

Cool-downs, on the other hand, keep your muscles from tightening up too quickly after you have completed your workout. By keeping muscles loose, both warm-ups and cool-downs help prevent injuries. If you move stiff muscles too vigorously, they will not give easily. Eventually tears form in the muscles or in the surrounding tendons that connect them to bone.

After completing the brief warm-up, you may begin the stretching and strengthening routine. The exercises first work the larger muscles of the lower body, further increasing circulation and preparing your body for the exercises that follow. The workout emphasizes the thighs, stomach and arms, which, in most people, are areas that require added flexibility and strength. Other benefits from the workout include improved co-ordination and reduced muscular tension.

The workout may improve your carriage and overall appearance by building up the muscles that contribute to correct posture. The push-ups and sit-ups included in the workout are among the best ways to strengthen your chest, upper arms, shoulders and abdomen. The workout demonstrates variations of these two exercises that range from moderately demanding to quite difficult. Choose the variation that is the most appropriate for your level of strength.

Interspersed with the strengthening exercises are stretches that will maintain the flexibility of the body areas being developed. During each stretch, you should push just to the point of resistance, relax slightly, then hold the stretch until the feeling of tightness diminishes, from 30 to 60 seconds. Do not attempt to stretch farther than you comfortably can. Stretching your leg muscles to the point where they begin to shake, for instance, could cause injury.

If you suddenly feel tired at any time during the 20-minute workout, stop and rest before you continue. Extreme fatigue may be a sign that you are exercising too strenuously and should slow your pace.

Breathe slowly and steadily as you perform the exercises. Holding your breath during strengthening exercises may produce erratic changes in your blood pressure, which will cause you to feel dizzy when the blood flow to your brain suddenly slows.

The aerobic activities demonstrated on pages 54-55 are just as vital to your fitness as the strengthening exercises. Performing a 20-minute

Workout Guidelines

◆ The key to strength-building exercises is to perform them steadily and with control. This will subject your muscles to relatively constant stress during both the lifting and the lowering phases. Above all, avoid quick, explosive movements, which can interfere with correct form and may also cause injury. During each exercise, move the joint involved through its maximum extension and flexion, or range of motion, to derive optimum strength benefits. (This also holds true for the flexibility benefits of the stretching exercises.) At the same time, be careful not to overextend or flex so far that the joint is bearing the workload: the muscles should do the work. No matter what type of exercise you perform, always work both sides of the body equally. If you stretch your left leg, for example, you should then do the same stretch with your right leg.

◆ Work steadily and evenly when stretching, taking care to avoid bouncing. Because it induces the contraction reflex, bouncing prevents the muscle from performing the stretch intended. It can also cause muscle tears. Exercise experts advise stretching a muscle only about 10 per cent beyond its normal length, which is the point where you feel tension but no pain. Flexibility cannot be rushed; if you are patient and consistent, you will see improvements.

◆ When exercising for endurance with aerobics, the most important factor is knowing how hard to push yourself. A simple rule of thumb is what exercise physiologists call conversational exercise: when working out aerobically, you should still be able to speak. If you cannot carry on a conversation because you are gasping for breath, you are working too hard. Conversely, if you can sing while you exercise, you are not working hard enough.

◆ If you have not exercised regularly for months or years, you may discover that some of the exercises in the 20-minute workout will cause muscle soreness within 24 to 48 hours — usually because they involve muscle groups that you have neglected. The soreness should subside in a day or two as your body becomes accustomed to the new demands on it. If the soreness does not lessen or disappear after two days, stop doing the exercises that aggravate the problem and consult a doctor.

aerobic workout three times a week will not only maintain your cardiovascular fitness, but it will also burn calories more efficiently than any other form of exercise.

Although the exercise routines in this chapter are called quick workouts, you should not rush them. The programme has been designed to give you full-body conditioning when you perform these exercises at an even pace — not at breakneck speed — for 20 minutes.

The 20-minute workout and aerobic exercises are not intended to replace longer, more intense workouts, but they can form the basis of an effective exercise programme. If you have trouble finding a convenient time and place to exercise consistently and regularly, combining these essential activities into a quick, efficient routine will keep you feeling fit and in shape.

Getting Started

Begin your workout with the warm-up exercises on these two pages, which should take two to three minutes. If you do the workout as soon as you get up in the morning, you should prepare for it by walking round the room for five minutes to wake up your body.

Warming up is important because it increases your heart rate, promotes blood flow to your muscles and prepares your tendons and ligaments for the demands of exercise. As a result, it makes the rest of the workout easier to perform.

Injury prevention is another of the benefits of warming up. While cold muscles tend to be stiff and relatively hard to contract, you can work warm muscles vigorously without undue risks of tears or strain.

Warming up also helps safeguard your heart. Studies show that three out of four people who engage in sudden, vigorous exercise without warming up exhibit abnormal cardiovascular activity, including irregular heartbeat. But researchers have found that warming up will prevent these problems, regardless of the exerciser's level of fitness.

After warming up, you will be ready to perform the strengthening and stretching exercises that begin on page 28. The routine first works the thighs and lower legs, then the abdominal muscles *(pages 34-39)* and concludes with exercises for the upper body *(pages 40-49)*.

The exercises combine stretching and strengthening activities. By alternating these two types of exercise, you will find the workout less fatiguing. The stretches will not only help speed your recovery from the more strenuous strengthening exercises, but they will also help your muscles remain loose and flexible as the workout proceeds. Hold each stretch for 30 to 45 seconds, except when otherwise indicated.

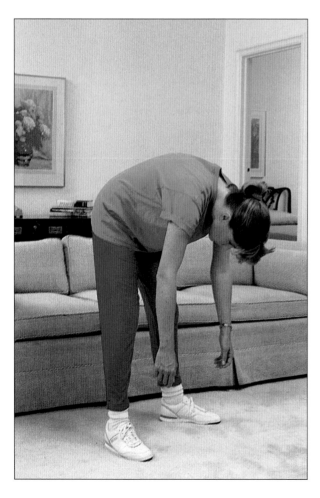
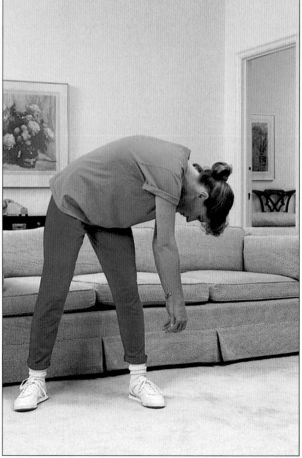

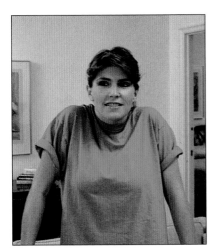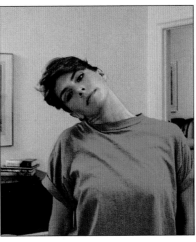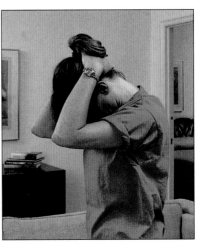

Stand with your arms hanging loosely at your sides. Shrug your shoulders, lifting them towards your ears five times.

Lean your head to each side five times, bringing your ear towards your shoulder without straining your neck.

Clasp your hands behind your head. Let the weight of your hands pull your chin to your chest and hold it there.

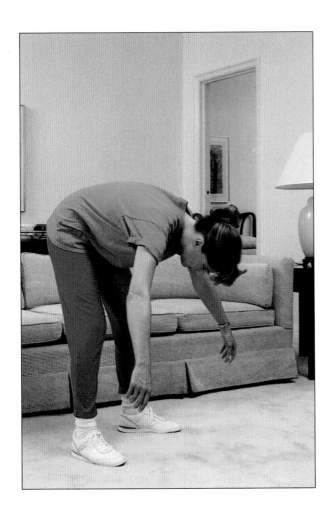

Standing with your feet spread about shoulder width apart and your arms hanging loosely at your sides, lean forwards as far as you comfortably can, keeping your head at waist level *(far left)*. Rotate each arm in a circle five times, alternating arms. Next, lean first to one side and then the other, and repeat the arm circles on each side *(centre)*. Then, leaning forwards once again, do 20 double-arm circles, moving both arms at the same time *(left)*.

Knee Press and
Outer-Thigh Raise

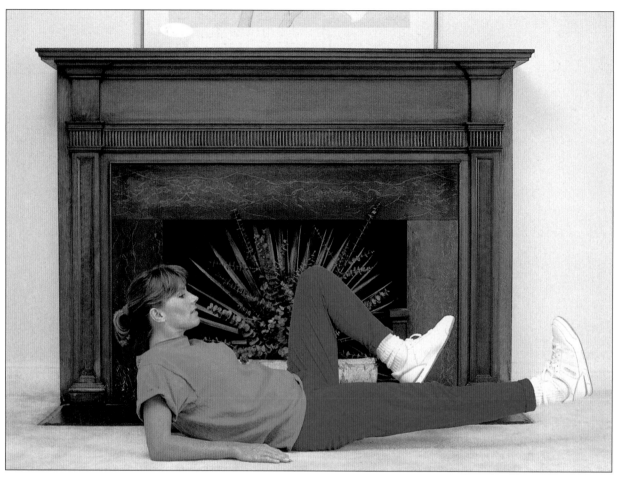

Lie on your back. Lift your upper body,
bracing yourself with your forearms resting
comfortably on the floor. Keep your legs
straight and your feet flexed. Bring one
knee towards your chest and lift the other
leg slightly. Straighten the bent leg and
bend your other leg. Perform the entire
sequence five times.

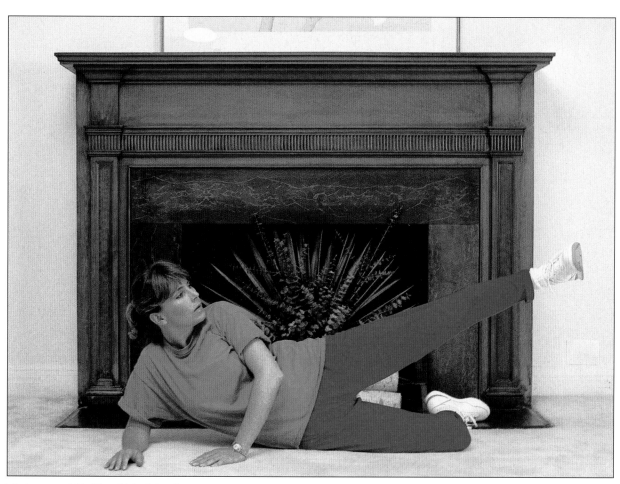

Lying on your right side, with both hands and your right forearm on the floor, bend your right leg to form a 90-degree angle. Keeping your left leg straight, flex your foot and raise the leg to about a 45-degree angle *(above)*, then lower it to just above the floor *(right)*. Do five repetitions, then turn over and repeat with your right leg.

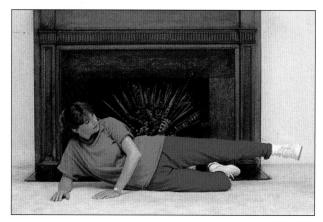

Inner-Thigh Raise
and Stretches

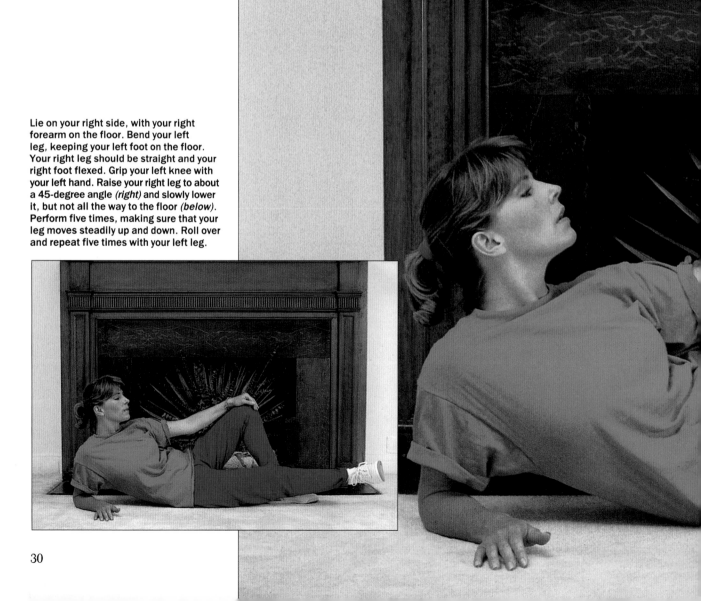

Lie on your back with your legs straight out. Prop up your upper body with your forearms, taking care not to overarch your back. Alternate bending each knee slightly, without lifting your heel off the floor. Perform five repetitions with each knee.

Lie on your right side, with your right forearm on the floor. Bend your left leg, keeping your left foot on the floor. Your right leg should be straight and your right foot flexed. Grip your left knee with your left hand. Raise your right leg to about a 45-degree angle *(right)* and slowly lower it, but not all the way to the floor *(below)*. Perform five times, making sure that your leg moves steadily up and down. Roll over and repeat five times with your left leg.

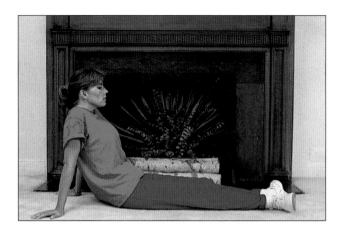

Sit on the floor with your legs extended straight out *(left)*. Place your hands behind you so that your weight rests on them; keep your arms straight. Rotating your ankles, slowly move your toes in a circle outwards as far as you can and then back to the centre. Do five repetitions.

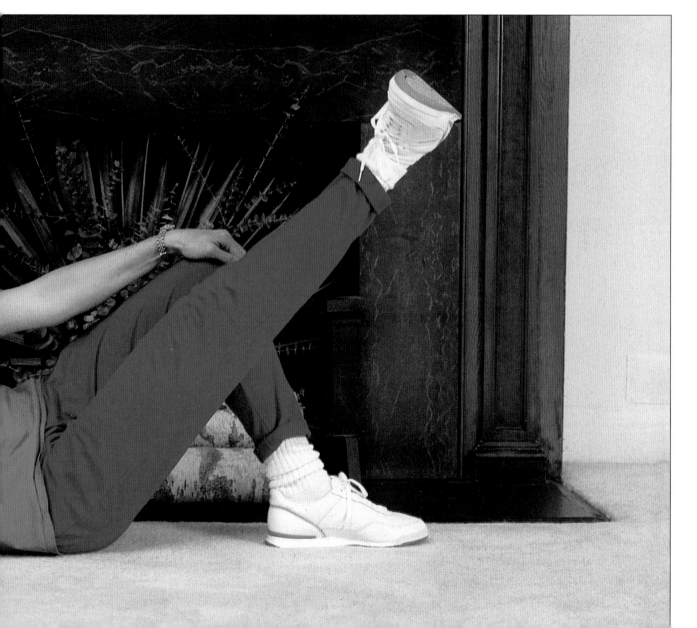

Thigh and
Hamstring Stretch

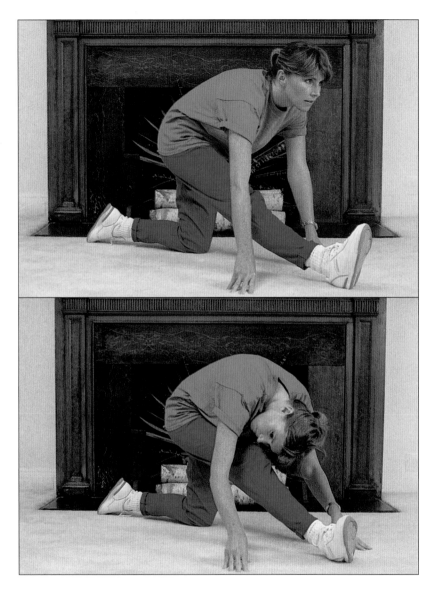

Crouch down so that your right leg extends in front of you and your left leg is bent behind you *(top, left)*. With your arms at your sides, bend your head towards your right knee *(left)* and hold. Switch legs and repeat.

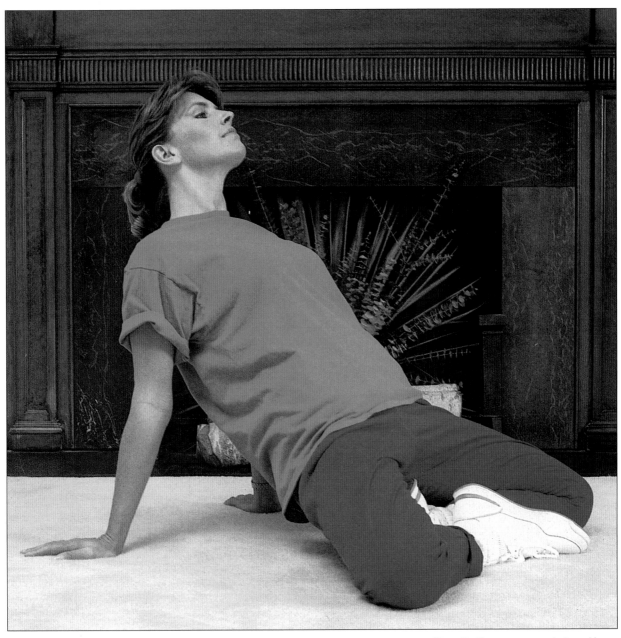

Sit on the floor, cross your legs and lean back slightly, supporting your weight with your hands. Gently arching your back, lift your lower body until you feel a slight stretch in your thighs. Keep your arms straight and lower legs on the floor. Hold.

33

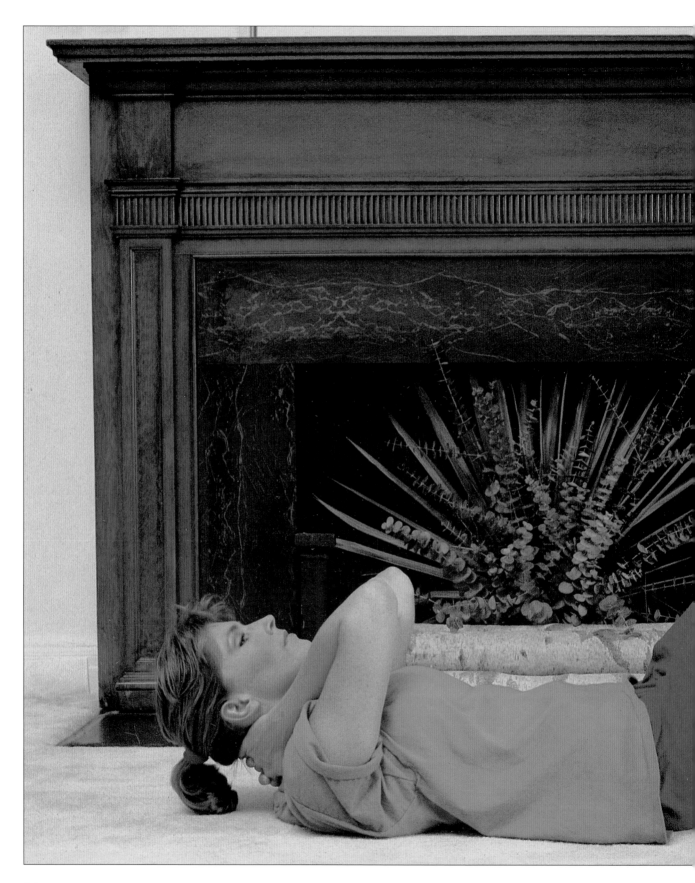

Stomach Curl

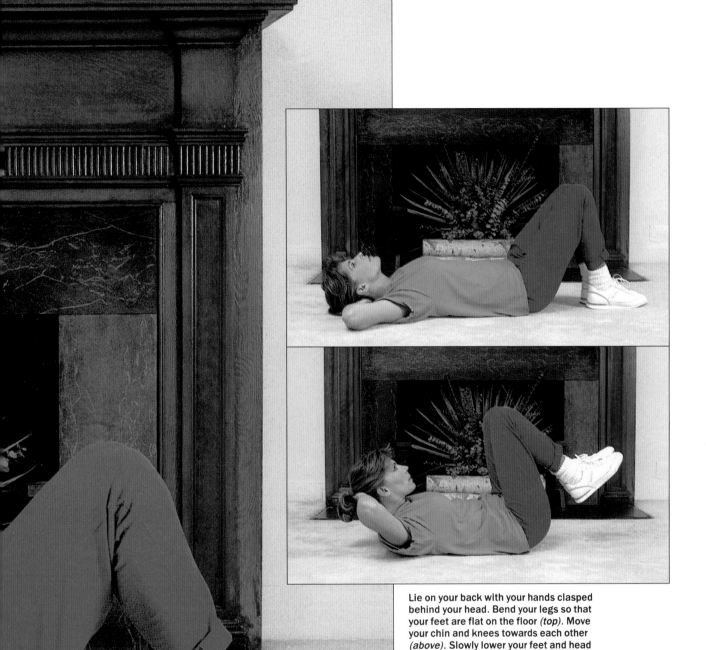

Lie on your back with your hands clasped behind your head. Bend your legs so that your feet are flat on the floor *(top)*. Move your chin and knees towards each other *(above)*. Slowly lower your feet and head back to the floor. Perform 10 repetitions.

Lie on your back, hands clasped behind your neck, knees bent and feet on the floor *(opposite)*. Pointing your elbows up, lift your upper body until your shoulder blades clear the floor. Slowly lower yourself back down. Perform 10 repetitions.

Hip and Back
Stretches

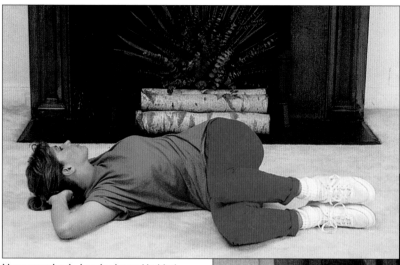

Lie on your back, hands clasped behind
your head, legs together, feet off the floor
(right). Roll your knees to the right as far as
you comfortably can and hold *(above)*. Roll
to the left and hold.

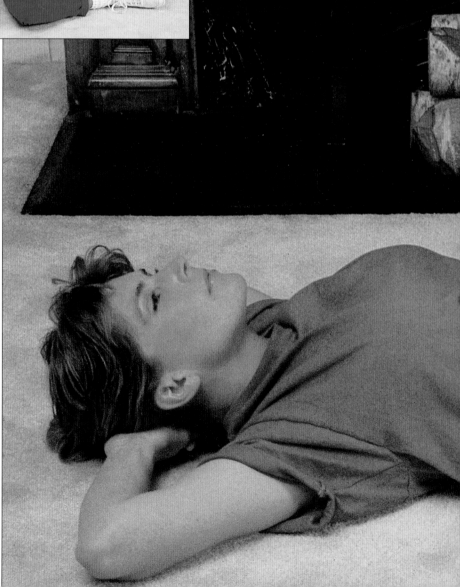

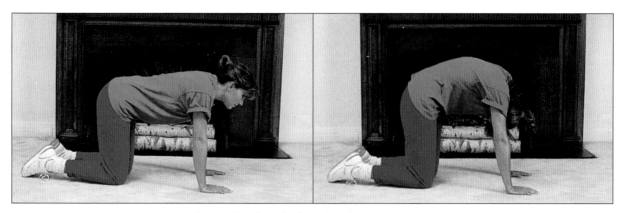

Get down on your hands and knees, placing your hands on the floor shoulder width apart, with your back straight *(above)*. Hang your head down while you round your back and hold *(above, right)*.

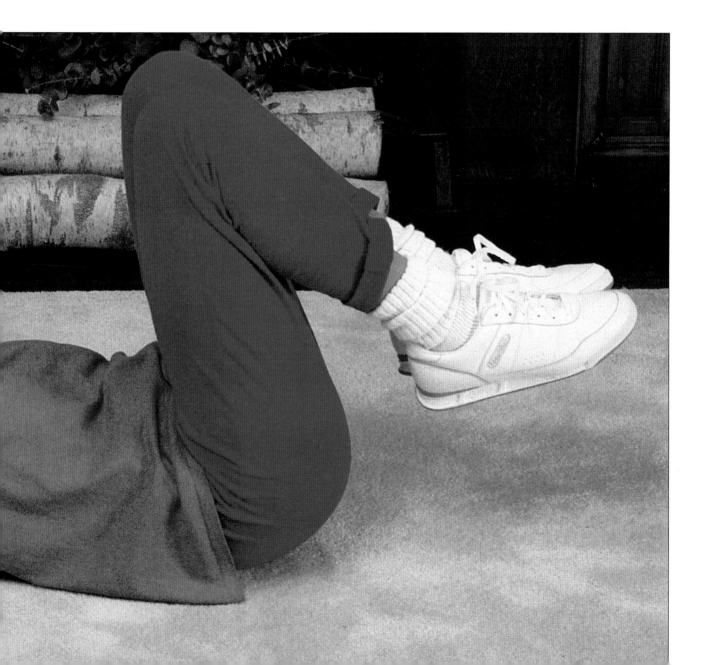

Diagonal Curl

Lie on your right side with your legs extended but relaxed. Bend your knees slightly. Cross your left leg over the right so that your left foot just rests on the floor. Point your hands towards your feet, your lower hand slightly off the floor *(opposite)*. Reach for your feet as you lift your upper trunk off the floor. Focus your effort on the muscles on the side of your trunk *(below)*. Slowly lower yourself back down. Perform the curl five times on each side.

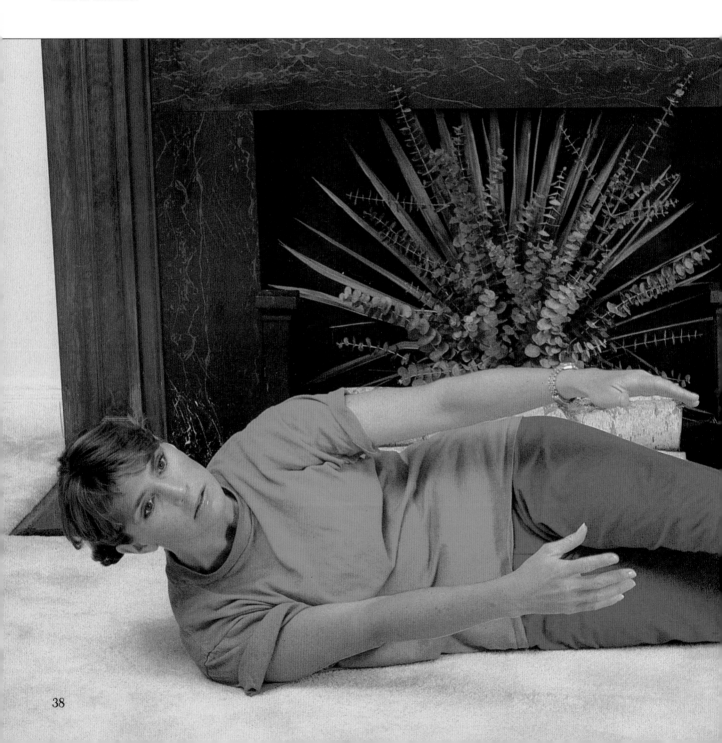

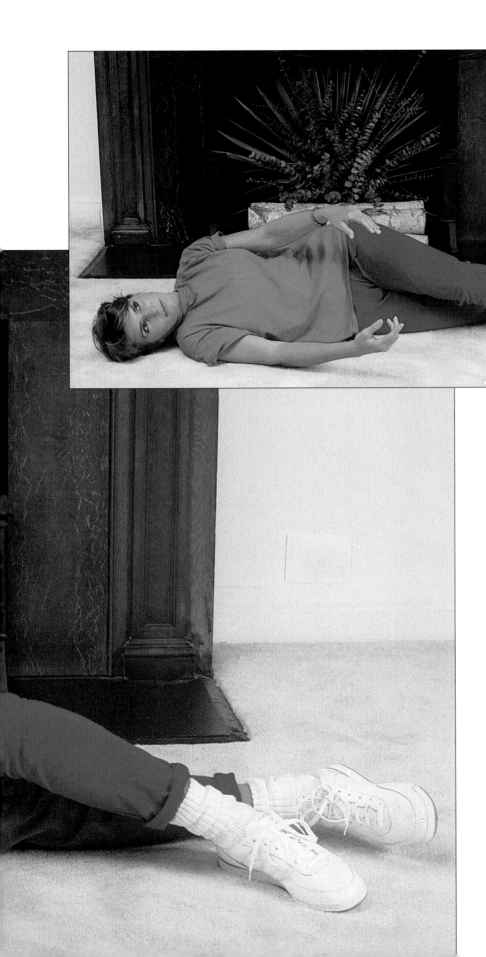

Push-Up
Variations

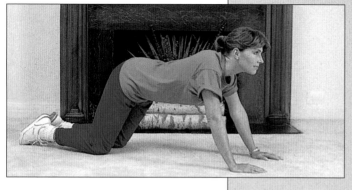

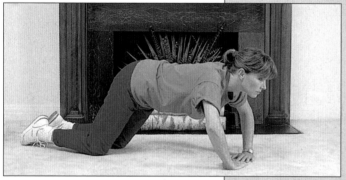

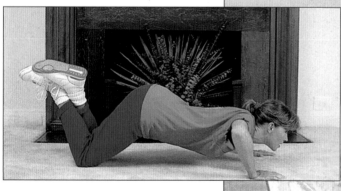

These versions of the push-up are of varying difficulty. In the easiest version *(top)*, begin on your hands and knees, placing your knees slightly farther back than your hips and your fingers pointing forwards. Bend your arms and slowly lower your chest to within 10 centimetres of the floor, then return to the starting position. Point your fingers towards each other *(centre)*, or cross your legs and lift them off the floor *(above)* to increase the effort. Do one of these push-ups or the more difficult classic push-up *(right)* five times.

Keeping your back and arms as straight as possible, rest your weight on your hands and toes. Bend your elbows and lower your chest to within 10 centimetres of the floor. Then raise yourself back to the starting position. Do five repetitions.

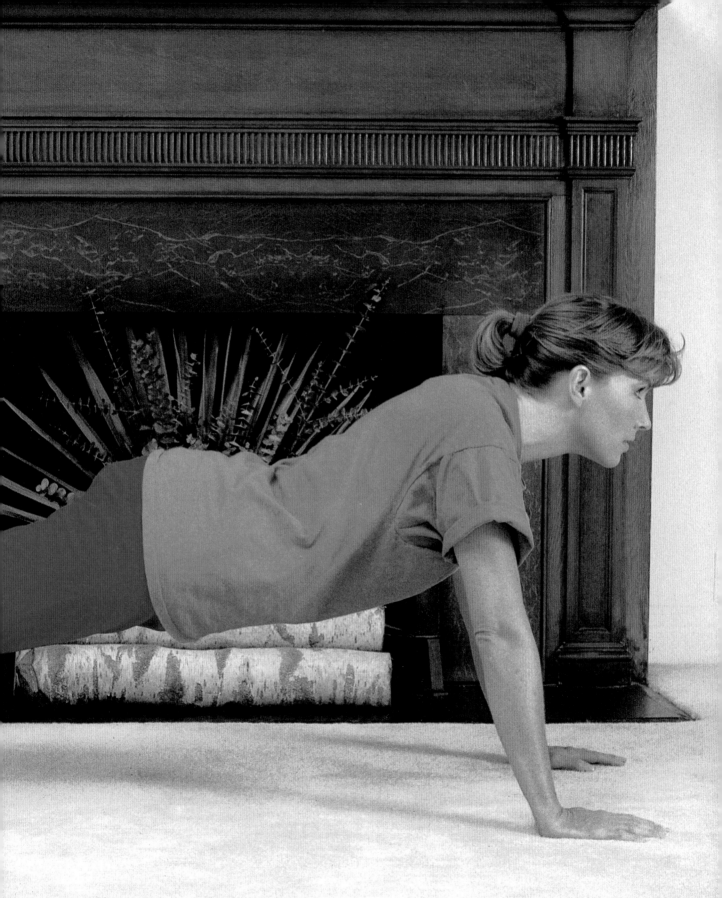

Upper Body Strengtheners

For developing the muscles of the upper body, it is necessary to supplement exercises for stretching and muscle-toning with routines that build muscular strength. Working with small weights is a convenient way to strengthen your arm muscles. You can also use certain types of furniture to help strengthen your muscles.

Furniture similar to the table used for pull-ups on this page and the chair used for dips on page 50 is readily available. However, the furniture you choose must be very stable; otherwise, it may fall over when you pull on it. The best choice for pull-ups is a sturdy desk or table. For dips and arm stretches a sofa is probably the best, most stable choice as long as you can grip it firmly.

A towel is also a useful piece of exercise equipment. In the 20-minute workout shown here, it is used mostly for stretching.

Weights may be the most difficult items to find if you are travelling. The best solution is to pack hollow plastic weights that you can fill with water; these are available at most sports-equipment shops. Alternatively, you can use books or other objects that weigh 1.5 to 4.5 kilograms (depending on how strong you are). The only requirement is that you can grip them easily.

If you do not have access to weights of any kind, leave out the weight-lifting exercises; instead, perform more repetitions of those exercises that develop the parts of your body that are the weakest.

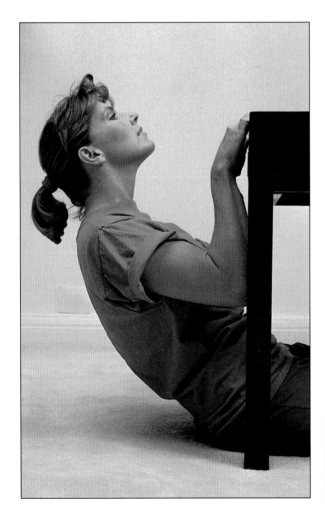

Lie down under a very stable desk or table, your hips flush with the table legs. Grip the edge and pull your torso up as high as you can; slowly lower yourself. Do three repetitions. Reverse your position so that your head is underneath the table and pull yourself up three times.

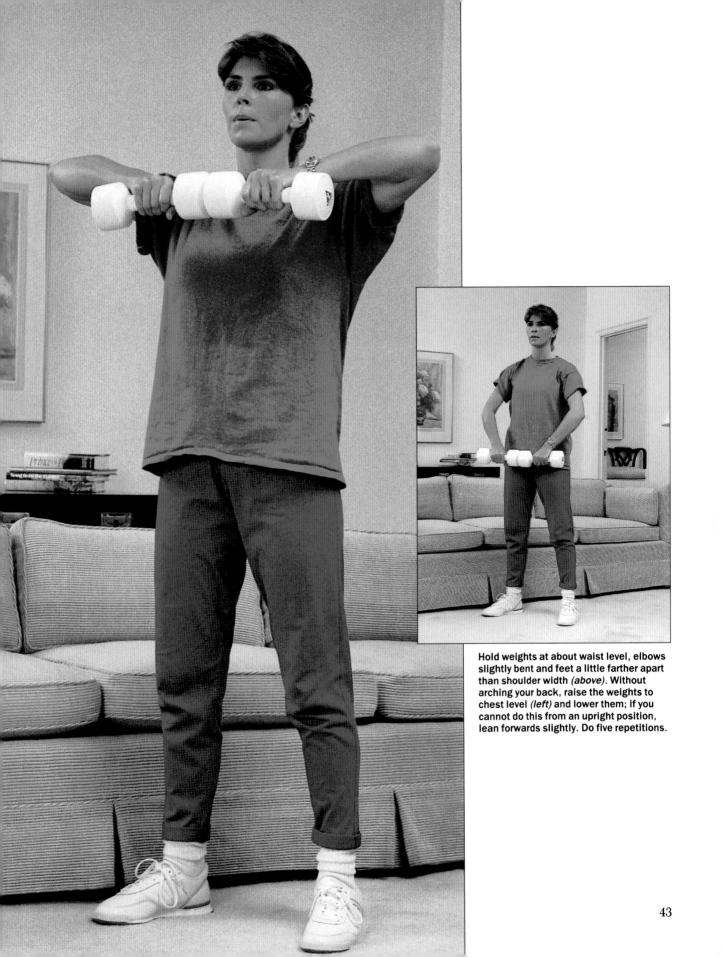

Hold weights at about waist level, elbows slightly bent and feet a little farther apart than shoulder width *(above)*. Without arching your back, raise the weights to chest level *(left)* and lower them; if you cannot do this from an upright position, lean forwards slightly. Do five repetitions.

43

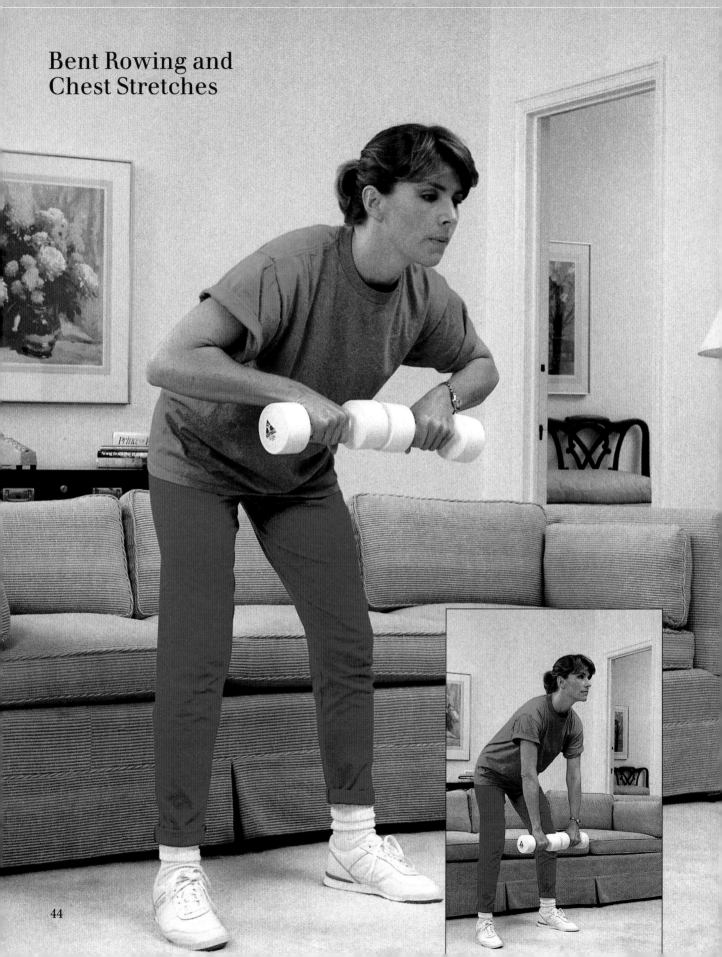

Bent Rowing and
Chest Stretches

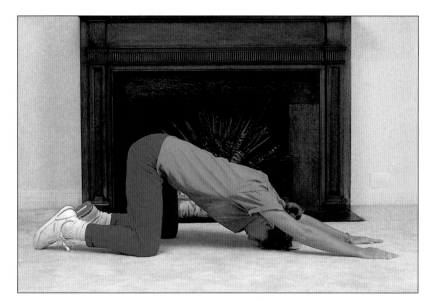

Crouch on your hands and knees. Put your hands on the floor and move them forwards as far as possible without straining. If you can comfortably do so, let your forehead touch the floor. Hold.

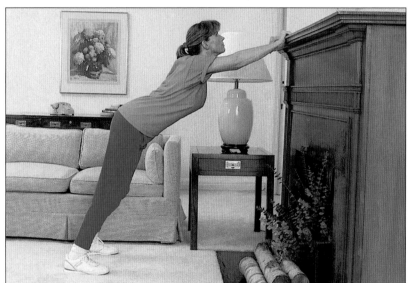

Stand about 1 metre from a stable piece of furniture. Grasp the furniture at chest level, then bend slightly from the waist. Keep your knees flexed and your back straight. Lean forwards and hold.

Grasp a pair of weights. Keeping your back straight and your knees bent, lean forwards so that the weights hang at arm's length *(opposite, inset)*. Do not lock your elbows. Bending your elbows and wrists, raise the weights as far towards your chest as you comfortably can *(opposite)*. Then slowly lower them to the starting position. Perform five repetitions.

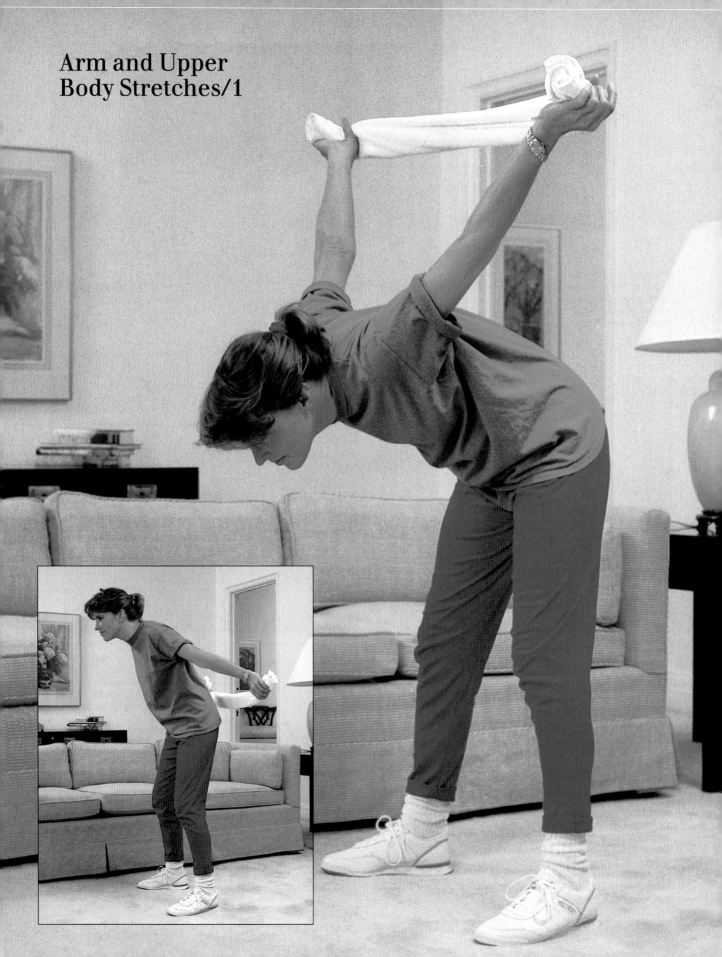

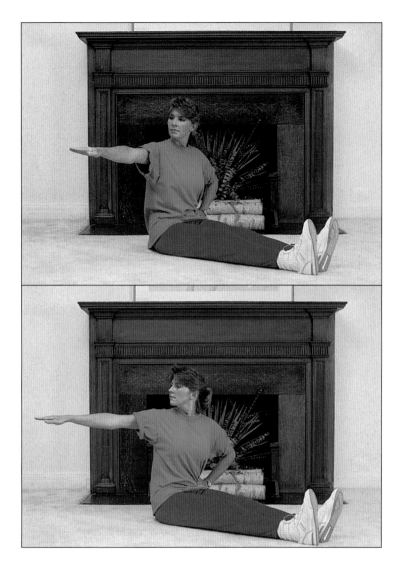

Sit on the floor with your legs outstretched. Place your left hand on your hip and extend your right arm to the side, with your palm facing the floor *(top)*. Moving from the waist, slowly rotate to the right as far as possible while keeping your arm straight and parallel to the floor *(right)*. As you turn, look over your right shoulder but do not force your head back. Hold and repeat on the other side.

Standing with your feet slightly more than shoulder width apart, hold the ends of a towel behind you and bend slightly from the waist *(opposite, inset)*. Lean forwards, bringing your head no lower than waist level, and raise the towel *(opposite)*. Hold this position and pull on the towel.

Arm and Upper Body Stretches/2

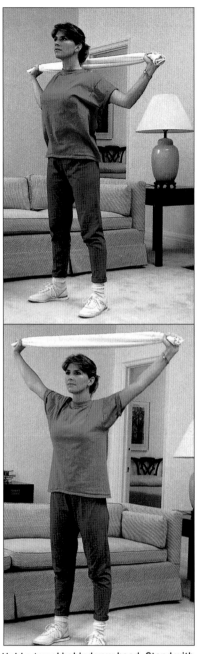

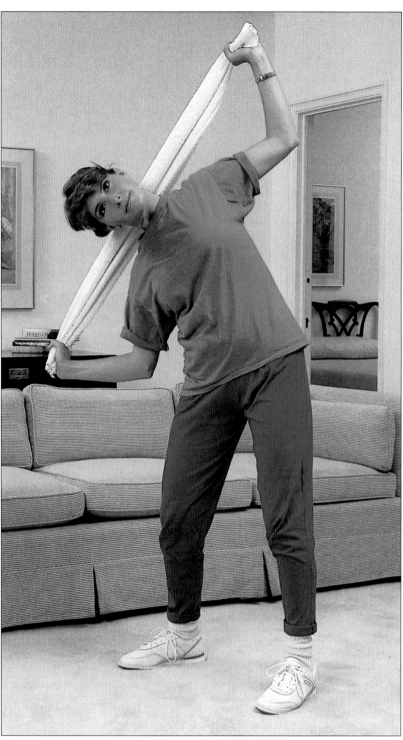

Hold a towel behind your head. Stand with your feet shoulder width apart and your elbows bent *(top)*. While pulling on the ends of the towel, raise it as high as possible and hold for a count of five *(above)*; lower slowly. Do five repetitions.

Holding a towel stretched out behind your head, lean as far to the right as possible and hold. Repeat on the left side.

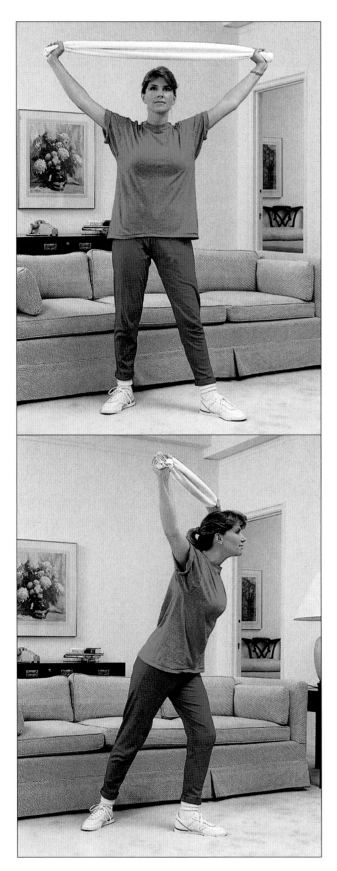

Stand with a towel stretched out overhead, your feet slightly farther apart than shoulder width. Without locking your elbows, pull on the towel *(top)*. Slowly turn to the left, shifting your weight to your left foot, which should be turned out to the left at a 90-degree angle *(left)*; most of the turning should be done from the waist. Hold and repeat on the other side.

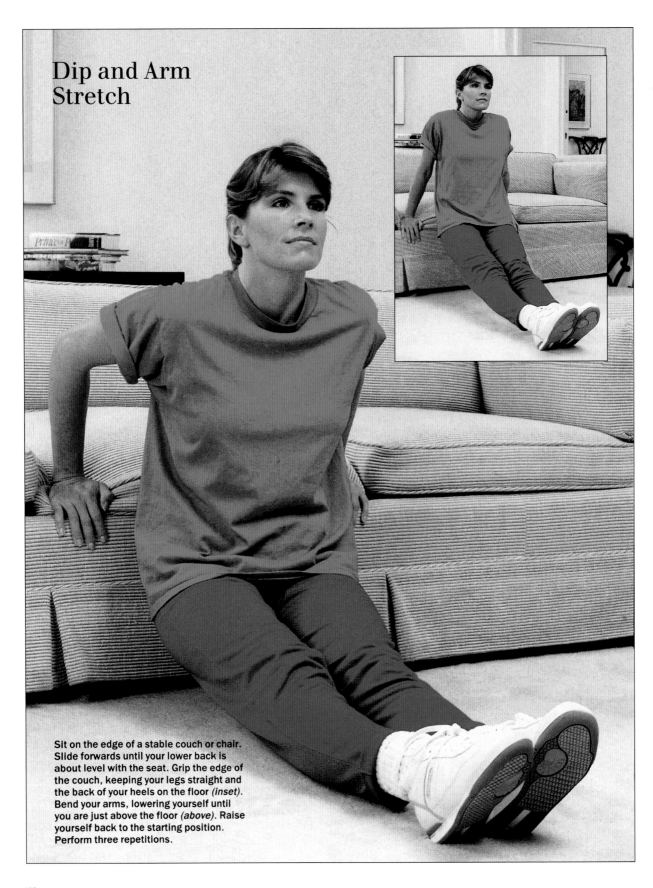

Dip and Arm Stretch

Sit on the edge of a stable couch or chair. Slide forwards until your lower back is about level with the seat. Grip the edge of the couch, keeping your legs straight and the back of your heels on the floor *(inset)*. Bend your arms, lowering yourself until you are just above the floor *(above)*. Raise yourself back to the starting position. Perform three repetitions.

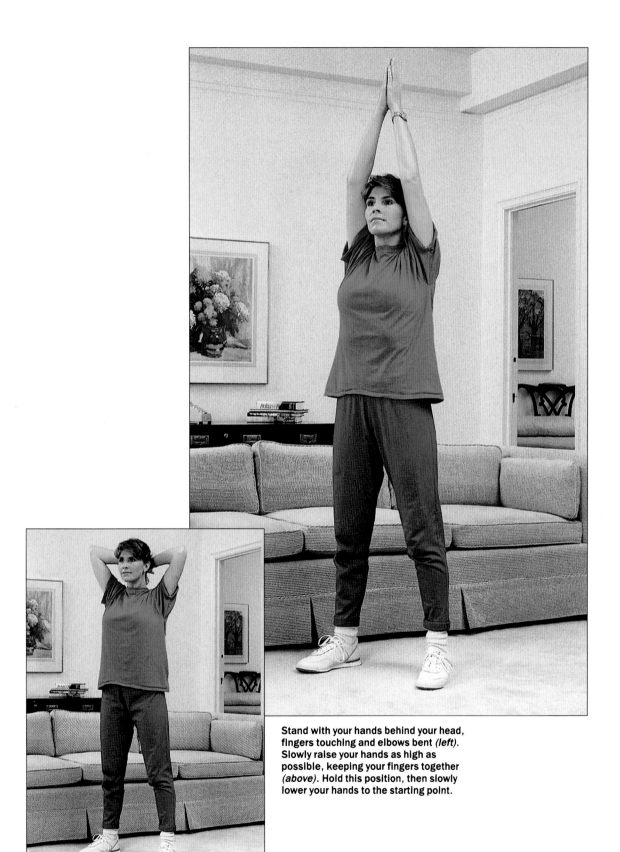

Stand with your hands behind your head,
fingers touching and elbows bent *(left)*.
Slowly raise your hands as high as
possible, keeping your fingers together
(above). Hold this position, then slowly
lower your hands to the starting point.

51

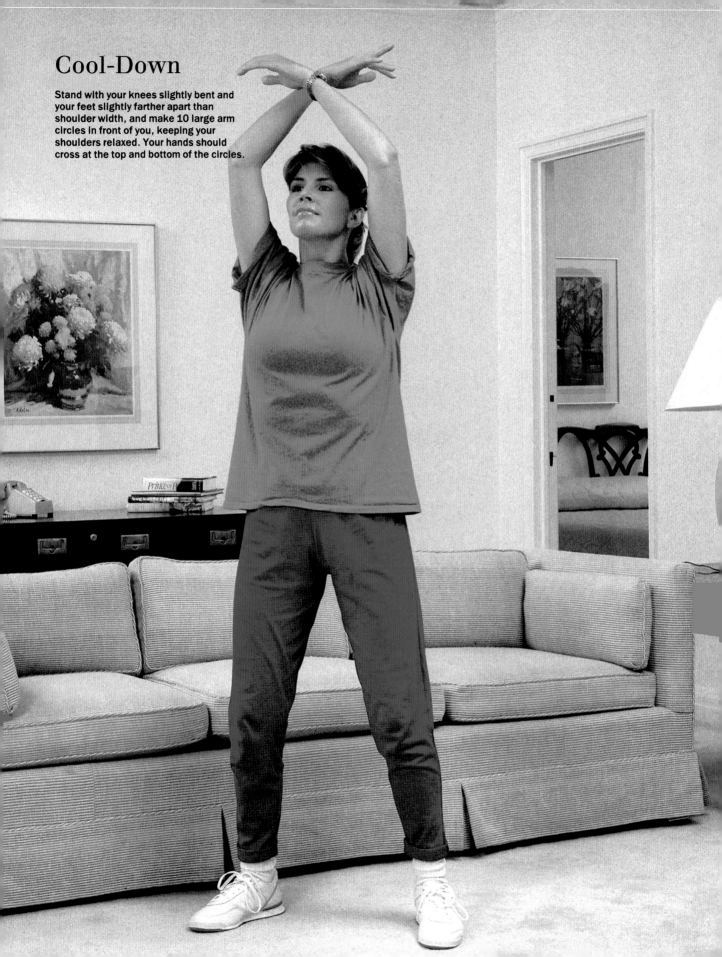

Cool-Down

Stand with your knees slightly bent and your feet slightly farther apart than shoulder width, and make 10 large arm circles in front of you, keeping your shoulders relaxed. Your hands should cross at the top and bottom of the circles.

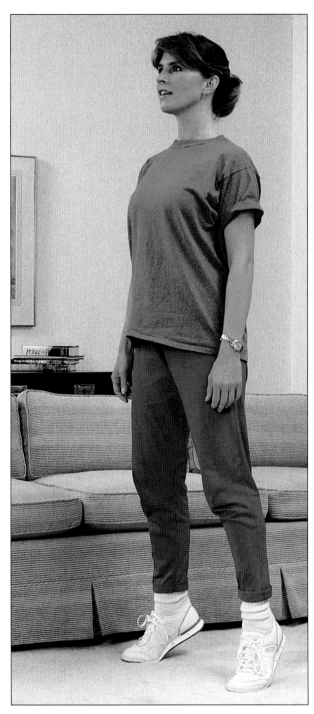 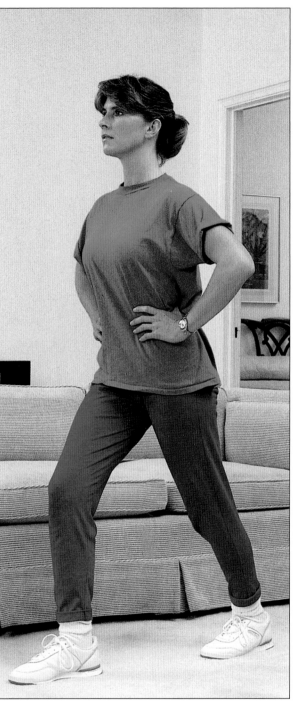

Standing with your arms hanging loosely at your sides, raise yourself slowly on your toes and hold for about two seconds. Keep your head straight and your shoulders loose and relaxed. Perform 10 repetitions.

Stand with your hands on your hips, your right foot forward, your right knee slightly bent, your left foot back and your left knee straight. Lean forwards until you feel a stretch in your lower left leg. Hold, then switch legs.

Indoor Aerobics

If you do not have access to a swimming pool, exercise bicycle or rowing machine, the most convenient indoor aerobic exercises you can do are running on the spot, jumping jacks and skipping. Although such activities are useful for increasing your cardiovascular capacity, they do place some degree of stress on your lower body and back. Proper footwear is therefore essential when you do these exercises. Never perform them barefoot or in worn-out shoes. Wear running or aerobic shoes that have adequate resilience. And, if possible, do your aerobics on a rug or padded surface. Women should wear a sports bra when doing these exercises.

To avoid boredom, do not limit your aerobic routine to one indoor exercise. For instance, you can start with seven minutes of running on the spot, switch to jumping jacks for three minutes, skip for three minutes and then return to running on the spot for the last seven minutes of your 20-minute workout. The warm-up and cool-down should consist of two to three minutes of any of these exercises performed slowly.

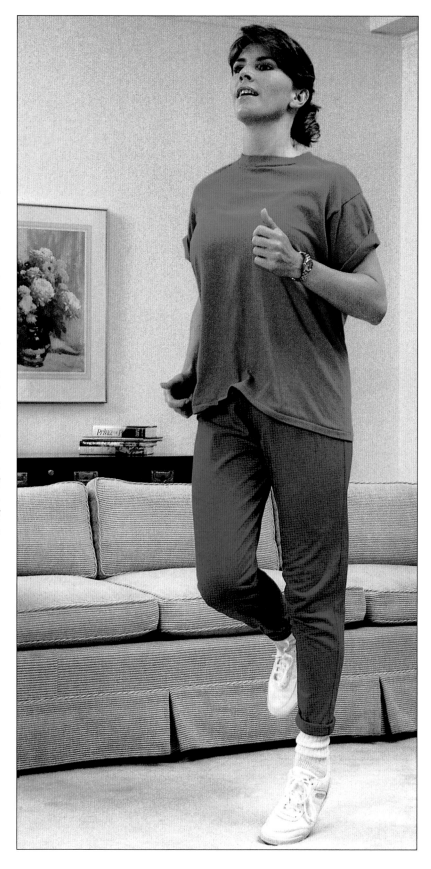

Run on the spot at a slow pace for two to three minutes, then pick up speed. Raise your knees higher to make the exercise more challenging. For variety, alternate running on the spot with moving around.

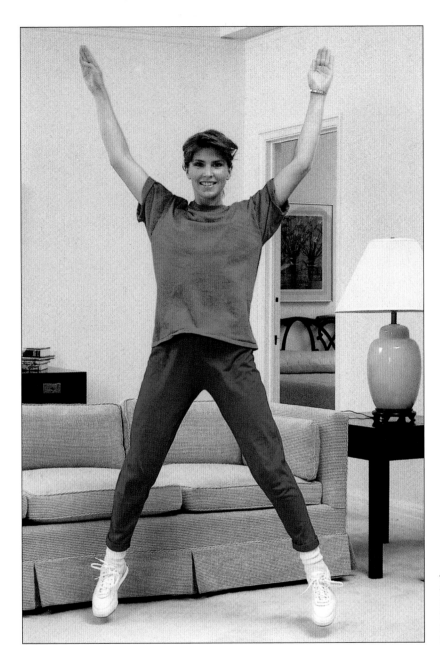

To do jumping jacks, start with your feet together and your hands relaxed at your sides. Jump up, moving your feet apart wider than shoulder width as your arms rise. Land with your hands over your head. Then jump again and resume the starting position.

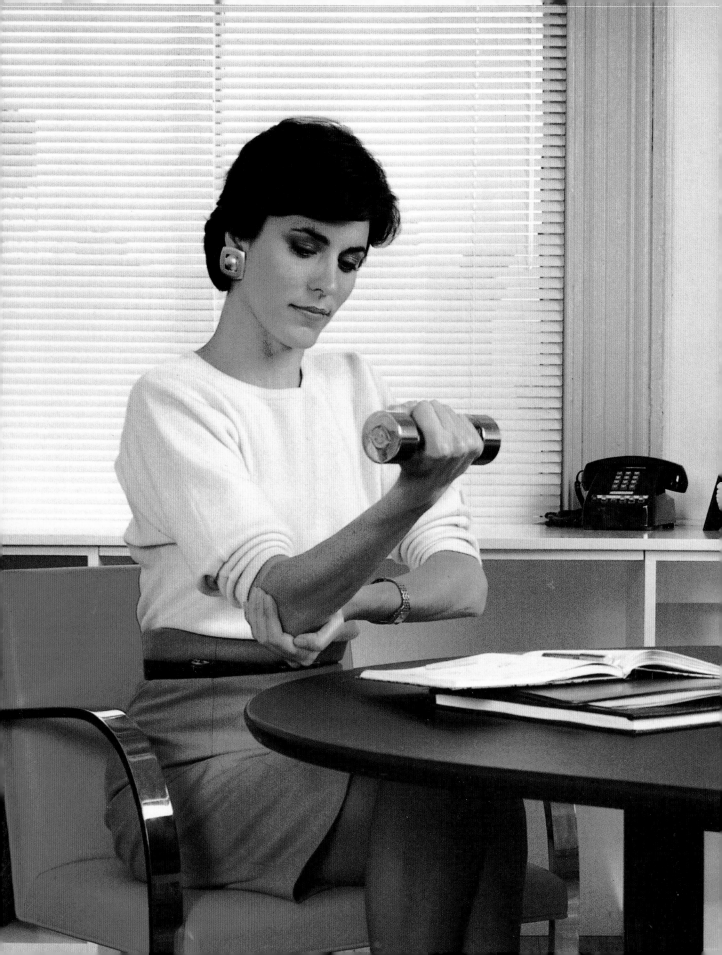

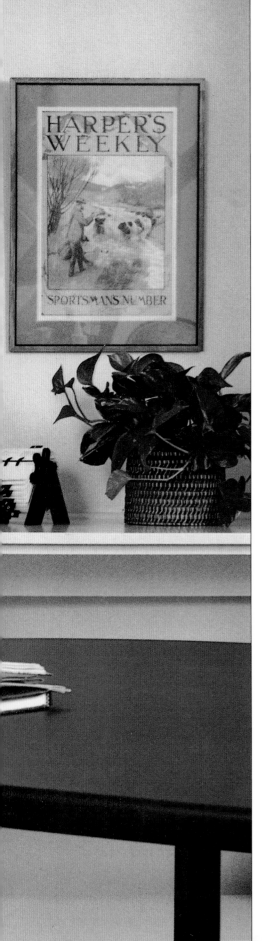

CHAPTER THREE

Office Workouts

Fitting exercise into your work schedule, stretching and muscle toners, aerobics at your desk

Sedentary employment distinguishes today's work force from those of previous eras: the vast majority of workers in Europe and the United States spend most of their day seated. Sitting for prolonged periods can adversely affect physical fitness in several ways. First, it contributes to weight-control problems by burning fewer calories than moving around or even just standing up. Second, long stretches of sitting weaken your stomach and back muscles; lower back problems are compounded by badly designed chairs or poor posture. Finally, sitting reduces the range of motion through which you move your joints. Desk work in particular restricts movement and deprives you of exercise.

Even if you do not sit all day, the chances are that your office environment and work schedule present little opportunity for getting sufficient activity, so that you must make a conscious effort to fit extra movement into your everyday routine. Furthermore, the conveniences of modern offices as well as the transport most people take to work tend to reinforce a sedentary lifestyle. Lifts, escalators, word processors, even push-button telephones may increase productivity, but they reduce the amount of physical activity in your life.

One way to compensate for not getting enough activity during office hours is to exercise before and after work. If you perform an efficient workout such as the one shown in Chapter Two and regularly walk, run, swim or engage in another aerobic exercise, you can tone your muscles and keep your heart in relatively good shape. But even so, you will still feel better and have more energy if you make a point of moving around and exercising during the working day. Studies show that some form of exercise, even if it is minimal, will improve your concentration, make you more alert and relieve tension. As a result, both your health and your job performance may improve.

The stretches illustrated on pages 60-65, for example, are excellent for retaining or restoring range of motion to your joints, and for preventing your muscles from losing their elasticity. Stretching is particularly important for those who work with electronic devices such as computer keyboards. It generally takes less effort to push computer keys than typewriter keys. In addition, a computer keyboard requires fewer changes in hand position: most of the time you hold your hands in the same place while only your fingers move. You may not move for long periods of time — you never have to change the paper, or even lift a pencil as you do if you are typing or writing longhand. As a result, when you work at a computer terminal for several hours at a stretch, tension builds up in your hands, shoulders and forearms, making you vulnerable to cramps or stiffness.

In addition, neck and back problems can arise from staring at a computer monitor or talking on a telephone for an extended period. The stretches included in this chapter can stimulate blood flow to your muscles, thereby relieving built-up muscular tension. The exercises emphasize bending and reaching in ways that most people tend to neglect during the typical working day.

Approach these stretches as carefully as you would any new exercise. Move into them gently and do not push yourself farther than you can comfortably go. Over several weeks, you will find that your flexibility will gradually improve as you become more experienced with the routines, and you will be able to reach and stretch farther.

Besides offering a setting for stretches, the office is also a good place for strength-building exercises. The exercises on pages 66-75 make use of both isometric and dynamic movements. Strengthening the upper body can be accomplished with isometrics that pit the arms against the hands, or with dynamic exercises that involve lifting books or other objects. Strengthening the middle body in an office chair usually requires swivelling while seated or simply tightening your abdominal muscles in an isometric squeeze *(pages 66-67)*; lower body exercises include shallow knee bends and thigh raises *(pages 68-69)*.

Your Work Space

◆ Many desks and chairs are designed in such a way that they can cause or aggravate such ailments as backaches, poor circulation and varicose veins. If you use a computer or typewriter at work, you may also suffer muscle problems in your arms, hands and shoulders. If you habitually tuck a telephone receiver between your shoulder and ear, you may find yourself with a stiff neck and upper back twinges at the end of the day. Interrupting your working day to take a walk — no matter how brief — or to do some of the stretches or other exercises in this chapter are the best ways to avoid or alleviate many of these problems.

◆ Try to set up your work space for comfort and efficiency. Make sure that the height of your chair is appropriate for your desk — and your body. Adjust the seat so that your thighs are parallel to the floor, your lower legs are bent at right angles and your feet are flat on the floor. (Another way to measure the adjustment is to stand up: the seat should be 5 centimetres below the crease at the back of your knees.) Your seat should not be so high that your feet dangle, nor so low that when your feet are on the floor, your knees are higher than your hips. At the same time, the back of your chair should firmly support your spine and encourage you to sit up straight. The back of the seat should tilt forwards and backwards, and it should be flexible enough to accommodate side-to-side movement.

◆ If you move around much while seated at your desk, make sure that your chair rolls easily. To roll with less friction on a carpeted floor, place a solid plastic mat under the chair's casters. An office chair with a five-pronged base is more stable than one with only four prongs.

◆ When working at your desk, you should be able to read material on the desk top without hunching over, and your bent arms should form right angles to your torso when you sit up straight. If your desk is so high that you must keep your forearms angled upwards, you run the risk of straining your muscles. If the desk top is too high and cannot be altered, raise your chair seat and use a footrest.

The aerobic movement routine shown on pages 76-87 offers another way to exercise at your desk. Although this routine is not as strenuous as running, swimming or cycling, it nevertheless burns calories, it can produce excellent aerobic benefits and it has the advantage of being a no-impact aerobic workout.

Performed sitting down, this routine is safer than conventional aerobic movements that call for jumping and bouncing, which can harm joints and bones. This routine is particularly beneficial for those who have not done any exercise in a long time, as well as for those who are seriously overweight and are not dexterous enough to perform aerobics that require a wide variety of arm and leg movements. In order to make this routine more enjoyable and to help you maintain a consistent pace, you can listen to music on headphones while moving through the sequence.

Office Stretches

Stretching exercises for releasing some of the tension that builds up during the working day can be done quite conveniently in most offices. You can do basic stretches for the upper body without even getting up from your chair. And you can perform stretches for the back and lower body while you stand next to your desk.

Relief of muscular tightness and tension requires awareness of the tense areas and conscious efforts at relaxation. As you stretch, remind yourself to loosen all tight facial muscles, straighten hunched shoulders and relax your neck and hands.

You can perform the stretches on this page and the following five pages at any time of day without being conspicuous. But if you feel self-conscious, you can disguise many of them by reaching for a book or a phone as you stretch. Letting a pencil drop to the floor, for instance, will give you an excuse to bend over, stretching to reach for your toes.

Do these stretches gently. For the first week or two, do not perform any of them more than twice a day, or you may injure muscles unused to being stretched. But once you are accustomed to them, you can do them as often as you like. Hold each stretch for 15 seconds to a minute.

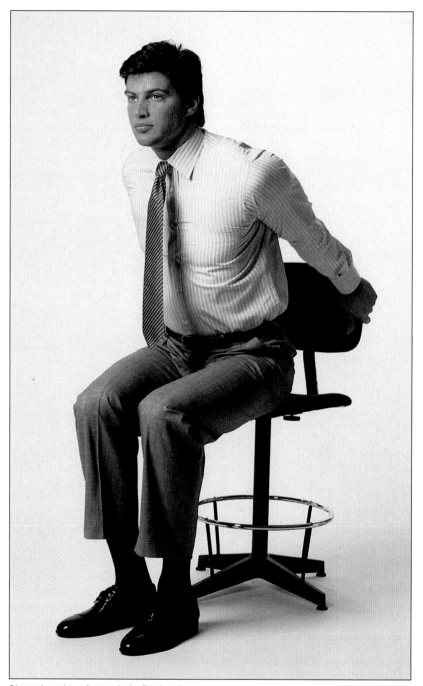

Sit on the edge of your chair, firmly grip the back and straighten your arms. Keeping your back straight, let your upper body gently pull you forwards to stretch your shoulders, upper back and chest.

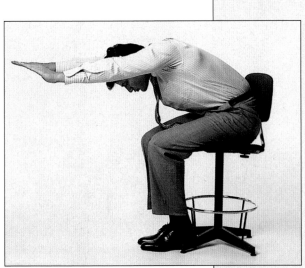

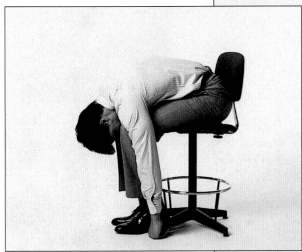

Reach up with your hands side by side *(right)*. Then reach forwards and down *(top)*, and move your hands apart. Keep your arms parallel to each other and let your chest fall forwards, your hands hanging at your sides *(above)*. Reach down as far as you can comfortably go but do not force yourself to touch the floor. Beginning this stretch with an upwards reach benefits the shoulders and upper back more than would merely reaching downwards.

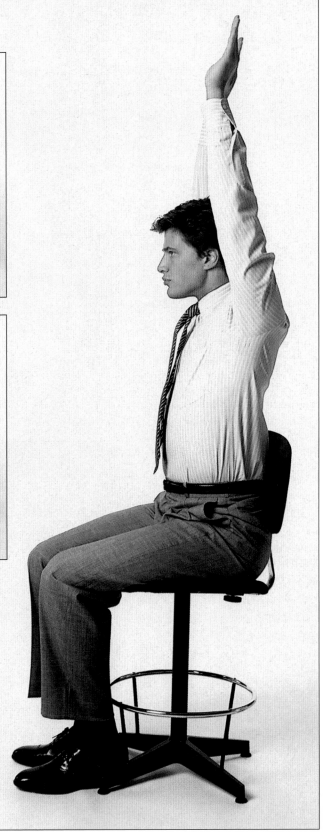

Shoulders

Reach up with one hand as you allow the other hand to fall towards the floor. Focus attention on the upper hand and imagine that it is floating gently upwards.

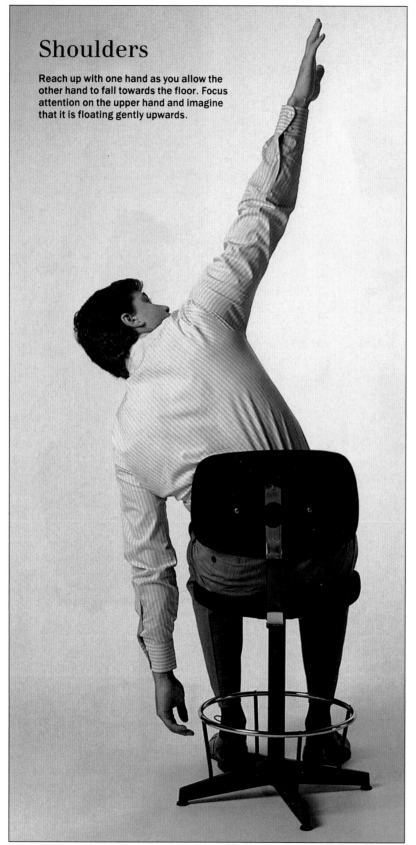

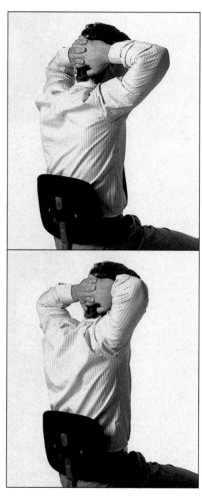

Sit upright with your hands clasped behind your head *(top)*. To stretch the upper back, gently pull your elbows back as far as you can and hold them in position *(above)*.

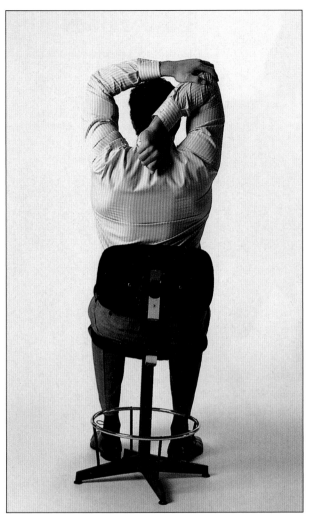 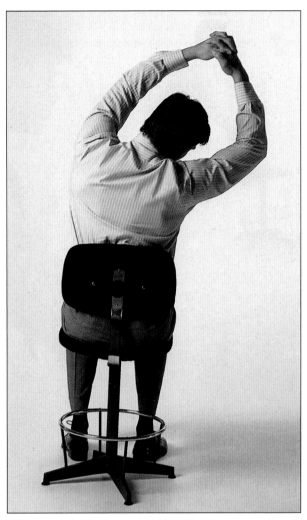

Clasp one elbow behind your head and pull down towards the back of your neck. Repeat with the other elbow. This increases flexibility in the shoulders and triceps muscle in the back of the upper arm.

With your hands clasped overhead, lean from your waist to the left and then to the right, holding the lowest position each time. This stretches the middle back and sides.

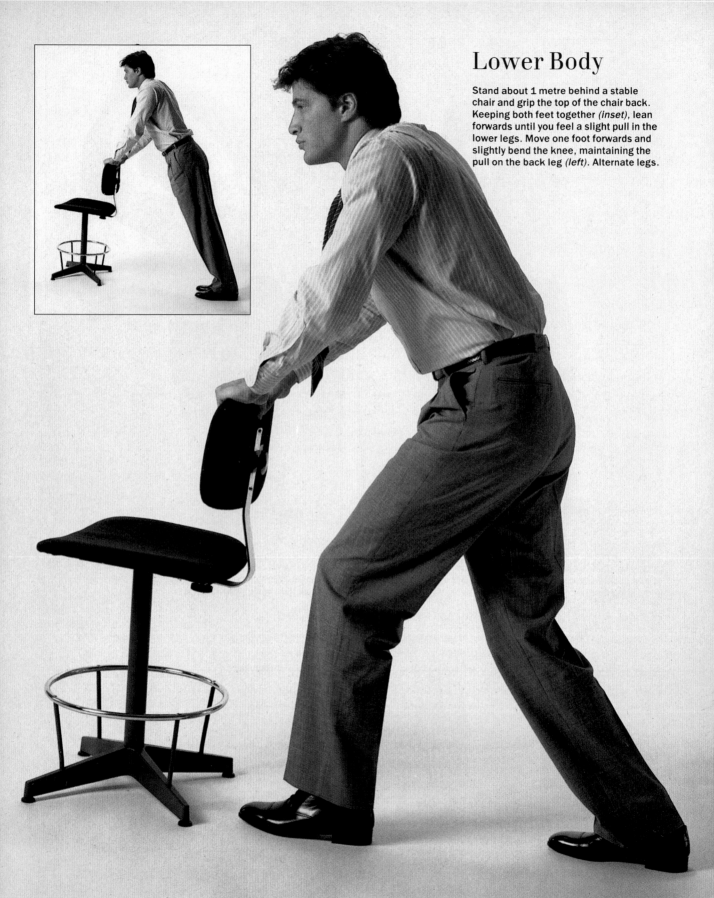

Lower Body

Stand about 1 metre behind a stable chair and grip the top of the chair back. Keeping both feet together *(inset)*, lean forwards until you feel a slight pull in the lower legs. Move one foot forwards and slightly bend the knee, maintaining the pull on the back leg *(left)*. Alternate legs.

With your right foot on your chair, place your left hand on your right knee and your right hand on your waist. Look over your right shoulder. Twist back as far as you can without straining, thus stretching the lower back and stomach muscles. Then stretch the other side.

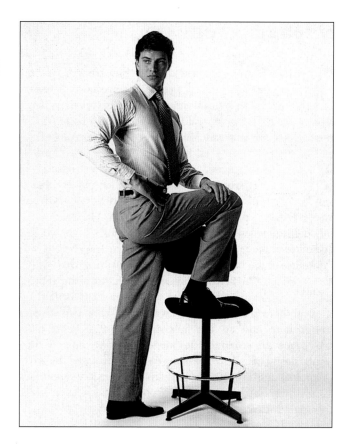

To stretch the upper leg, stand about 30 centimetres from your chair and place the instep of your right foot on the chair seat. Bend your left leg slightly until you feel a gentle stretch in the top of the raised leg. Repeat with the other leg.

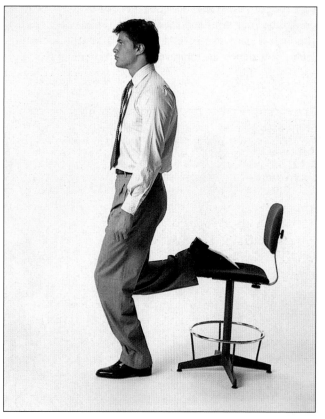

Strengtheners

There are two basic ways to do dynamic strength exercises in the office: you can either do variations on simple callisthenic movements, or you can lift readily available objects such as books or paperweights. Vigorous, prolonged callisthenics, or aerobic movements, provide benefits for cardiovascular conditioning, and lifting objects not only helps develop strength, but also shapes and tones muscles.

Because of the limited space in the workplace and the restraints on your movement, the callisthenics you can perform there are restricted. The exercises here and on the following two pages are confined to movements designed to strengthen your abdominal and lower body muscles. All of them can be done while you are seated except for the shallow knee bends *(page 69)*.

The exercises in which books are used *(pages 70-73)* are designed to strengthen your arms and shoulders. Although it may take several weeks before you notice an improvement, the strength you develop from these exercises will make it easier for you to carry your luggage and bags of groceries, and to play racket sports with more power.

The first time that you perform these exercises, be careful not to select objects that are too heavy for you. Always err on the side of caution, at least until the exercises are comfortable and familiar. Begin with five repetitions of each exercise, ensuring that you perform each exercise to the right as many times as you do to the left.

When you are ready to make these exercises more difficult, you can lift heavier objects. Be careful, though, to increase the weight slowly: this is especially important for those who have, or have previously had, back problems. When you are no longer able to increase the weight because of the limited number of objects available in your office, you can advance to a more challenging level by gradually increasing the number of repetitions that you do.

Keeping your chin up and your back as straight as you can, grip your chair *(below, left)* and lift your legs *(centre)*. If you feel a pull in your lower back, your legs are too high and you should lower them. Swivel your legs to alternate sides *(below)* to include the side abdominal muscles. Lifting your knees towards your chest contracts the abdominal muscles and also strengthens the quadriceps, which are the muscles on the front of your thighs.

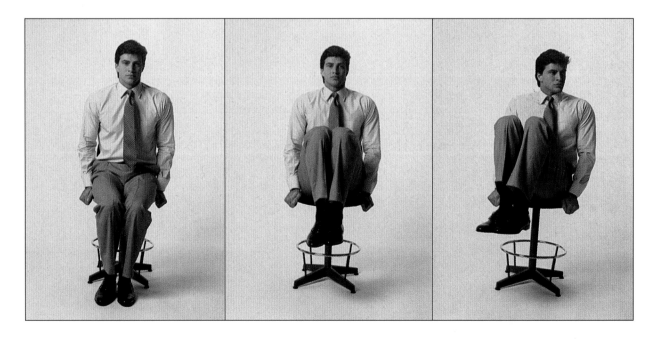

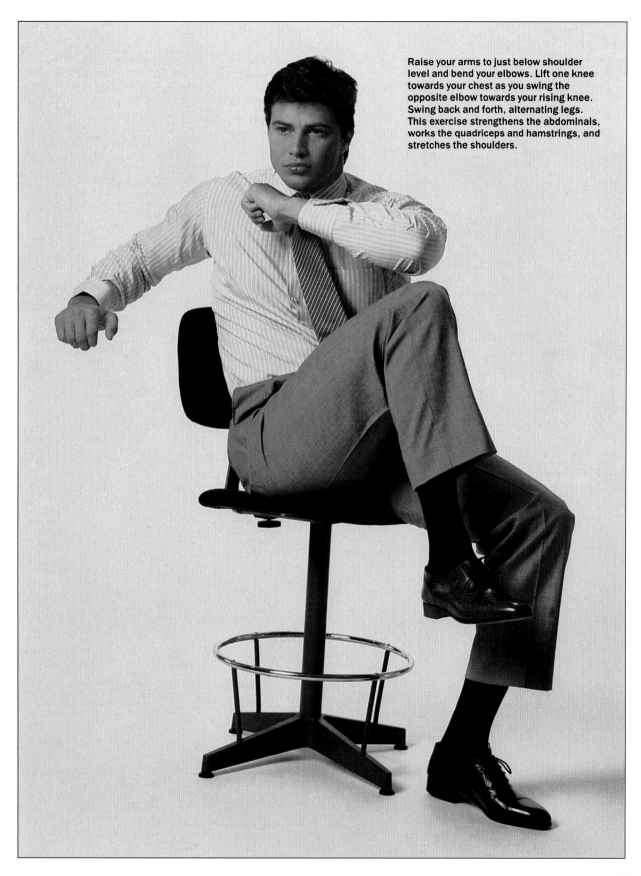

Raise your arms to just below shoulder level and bend your elbows. Lift one knee towards your chest as you swing the opposite elbow towards your rising knee. Swing back and forth, alternating legs. This exercise strengthens the abdominals, works the quadriceps and hamstrings, and stretches the shoulders.

Legs

Sit down, grip the seat of your chair and raise one leg while you flex your foot *(left)*. Slowly move your leg outwards *(inset)*, then back towards the centre and down. This will tone your thighs.

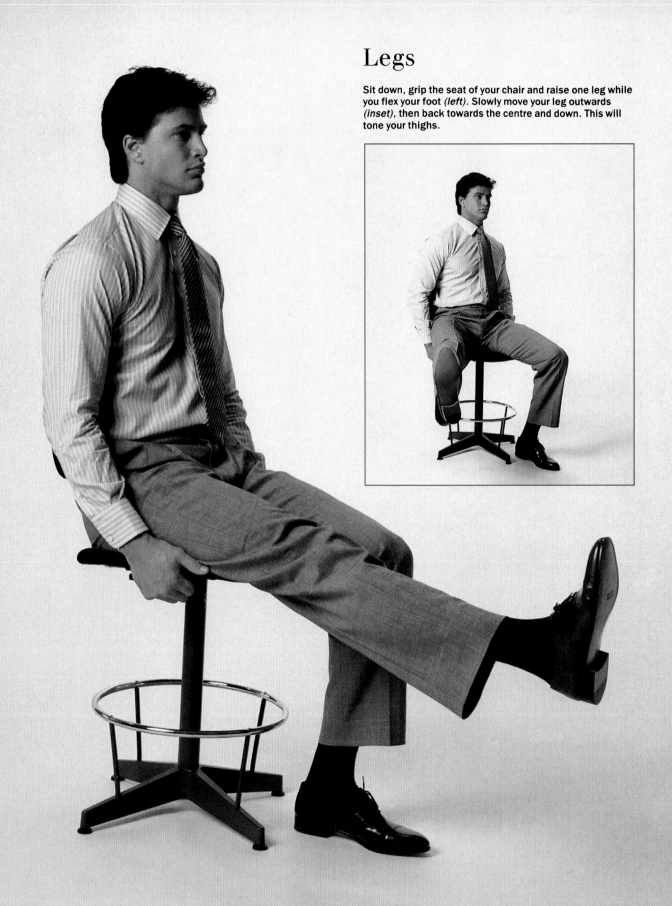

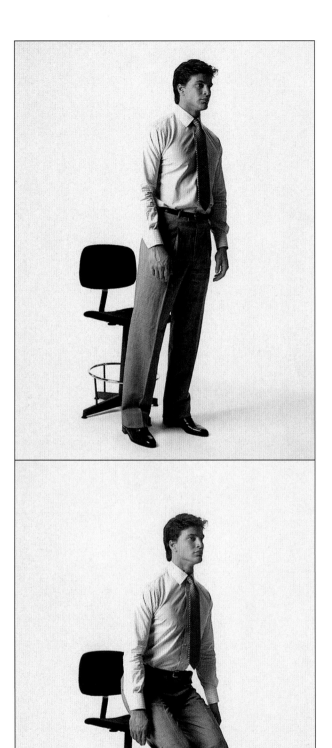

Do a shallow knee bend for your upper legs. Stand up with your back straight *(top)*. Bend your knees but not so far that your buttocks drop below knee level *(bottom)*.

Arms/1

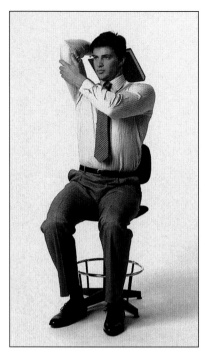

To increase strength in your triceps, sit down and, holding a book in one hand, reach behind your shoulder; keep your palm facing up and the opposite hand supporting your elbow *(above)*. Raise the book until your arm is straightened *(right)* and then slowly lower your arm to the starting position.

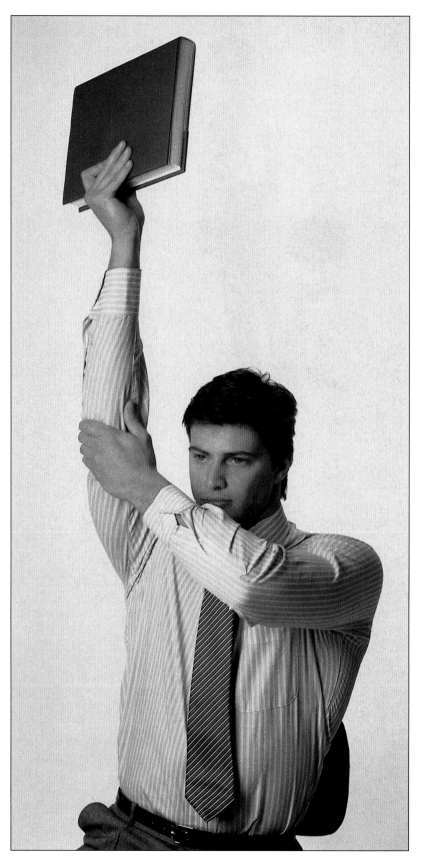

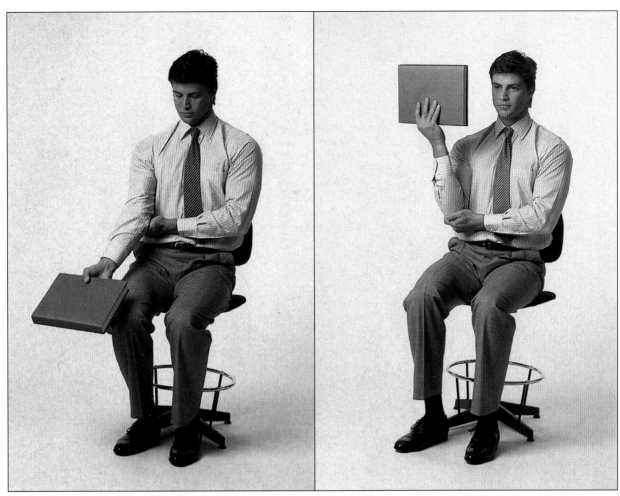

With your palm up, hold a book level with your knee. Use the
opposite hand to support your elbow *(above)*. Raise the book to
your shoulder *(right)* and then lower it, working your biceps.

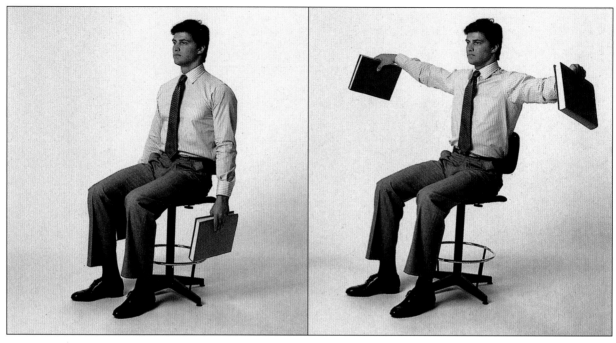

To work the shoulders, start with a book in each hand and let your arms hang down *(above)*. Keeping your arms straight at all times, lift them to shoulder height *(right)*.

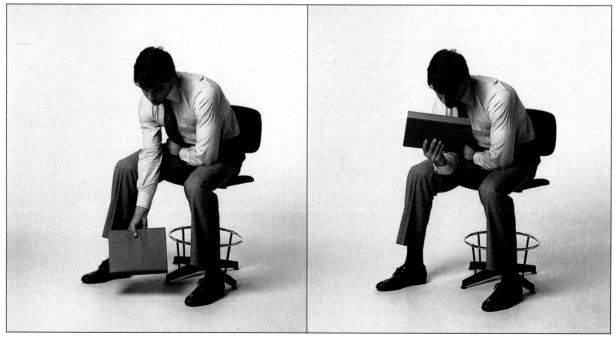

Hold a book in one hand. Lean over and dangle it between your legs with your arm straight *(above)*. Then lift the book to your chest *(right)*, keeping your elbow on your upper leg.

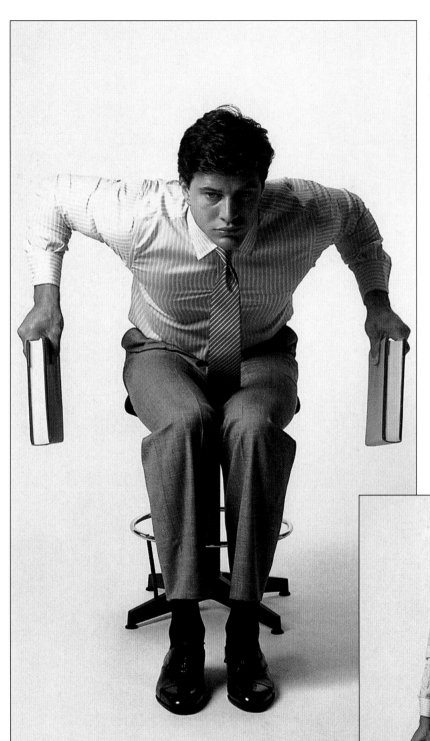

Lean forwards with books in both hands at your sides, keeping your arms extended *(below)*. Bend your elbows to lift your arms, bringing the books to chest level *(left)*. Lower the books and repeat nine times. This motion works the triceps and shoulder and upper back muscles.

Isometrics

The most convenient exercises for building strength in the office are isometrics, which require no equipment and can be done unobtrusively at your desk. To do isometrics, you tighten a muscle without moving your body. As you do so, you are toning a pair of opposing muscles, since it is almost impossible to tighten a single muscle and remain still unless something opposes that muscle's motion.

For instance, if you tighten the biceps without moving, your triceps also tightens. (You can feel your tightened triceps, the muscle on the back of your upper arm, with the hand of your other arm.) If your triceps stayed relaxed, your forearm would move upwards. If, however, you tighten the biceps by pushing your hand up against an immovable object such as your desk, the triceps stays relatively relaxed, because the desk restricts the arm's motion.

Whenever you perform isometrics, you should maintain steady breathing. Some people have a tendency to hold their breath as they push hard, striving for a maximal muscle contraction. This is a mistake that can cause dizziness by interfering with your circulation.

Each isometric contraction should be held for five to 10 seconds, and should be done an equal number of times on both sides. To build strength, each exercise should be done three or four times daily, and at several different angles. Perform any neck exercises gently at first to avoid possible injury.

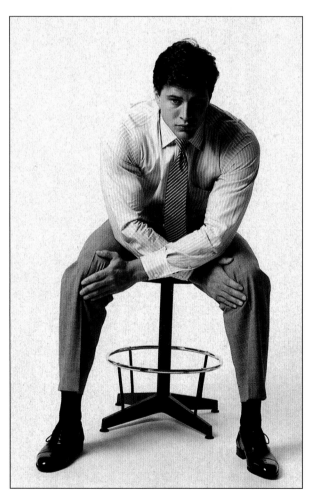

To tone your arms and lower back, lean forwards with your legs apart; push with your hands on the insides of the opposite knees.

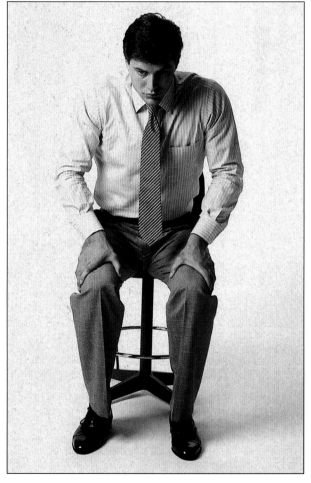

Push down with your hands on your upper thighs to strengthen your triceps and upper back muscles.

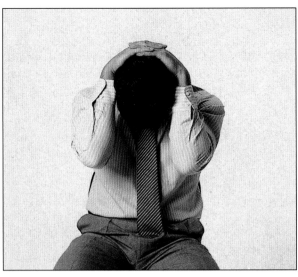

To tone your forearms and neck, clasp your hands behind your head, drop your chin to your chest and push your head up against your hands.

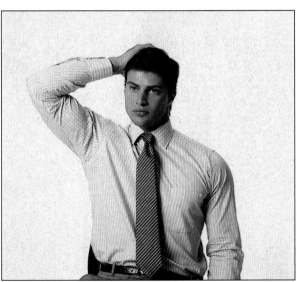

With one hand on the side of your head, push sideways, opposing the motion with your head. This strengthens your neck and shoulder muscles. Alternate sides.

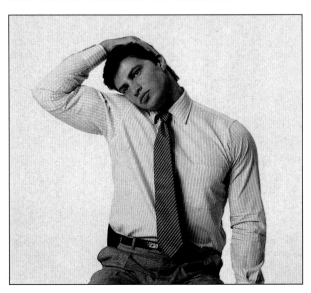

Reach over the top of your head and pull down your hand, opposing the motion with your head to develop the muscles of your forearms and neck. Alternate sides.

Aerobics/1

Any prolonged and rhythmic movement that increases the muscles' demand for oxygen and nutrients carried by the blood is a form of aerobic exercise. Because the extra demand for circulating blood makes the heart work harder, when you perform aerobic exercise regularly your heart adapts to the workload, increasing its capacity to meet the demand.

Performing aerobic movements does not mean that you have to spend an hour running around a track or jumping up and down in specially designed shoes and clothes. In fact, you can raise your heart rate just by moving round unobtrusively in your office chair.

Among the exercises shown on these and the following 10 pages are routines called jarming, which involve only arm movements. Some companies that organize daily exercise breaks for their employees use jarming to help office workers relieve their stress and boredom. By increasing circulation to your arms and upper body, a few minutes of jarming can make you more alert and help fight the cramps and muscle tightness that can occur after a long period of sitting.

When you exercise in your chair, you will find that the movements that involve lifting your arms over your head and swinging your feet simultaneously are the most effective at increasing the rate at which your heart pumps blood. As you run through the routine, devote about a minute to each movement.

Begin your aerobic workout with gentle upward reaches, alternating hands.

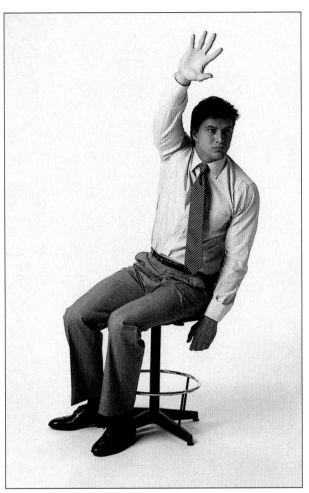

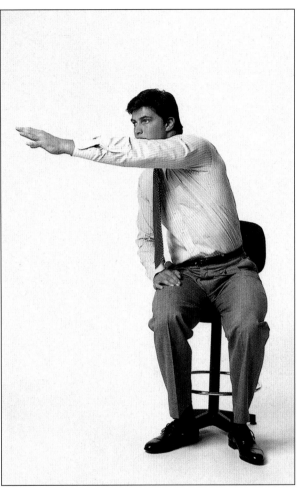

Gradually shift from reaching straight up towards the ceiling to reaching sideways, across your body at an angle, alternating arms. Keep your hands loose and relaxed.

Reach across your body, alternating arms but keeping them approximately parallel to the floor at shoulder height. Let your weight shift back and forth in the direction of your reach.

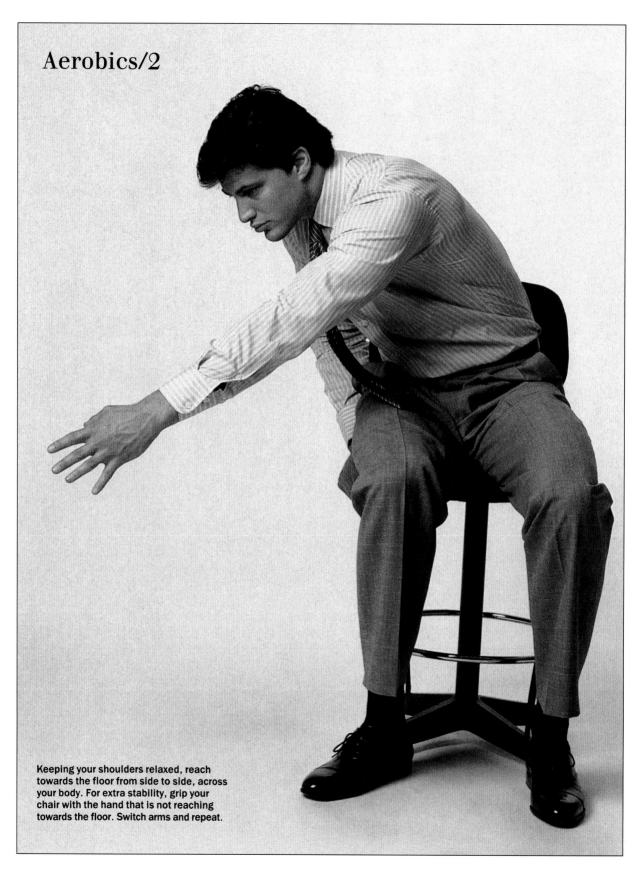

Keeping your shoulders relaxed, reach towards the floor from side to side, across your body. For extra stability, grip your chair with the hand that is not reaching towards the floor. Switch arms and repeat.

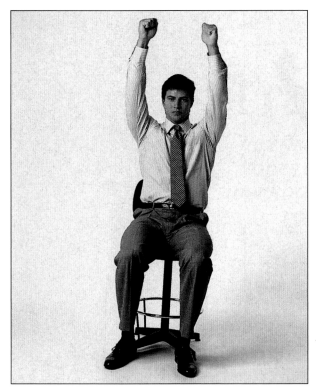

Flex your arms so your hands, in loose fists, almost touch your shoulders. Reach up and down, arms in unison.

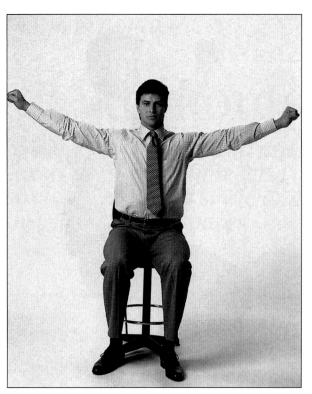

Start again with bent elbows. Reach your fists out to the side, keeping the hands slightly above shoulder height.

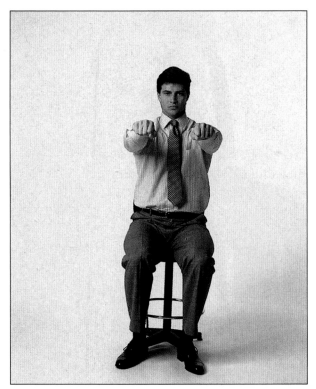

With your palms facing down, move your fists in and out in front of you by bending and straightening your elbows.

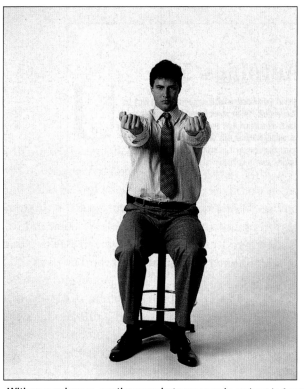

With your palms up, continue moving your arms in and out in front of you. As they come towards you, flare your elbows out.

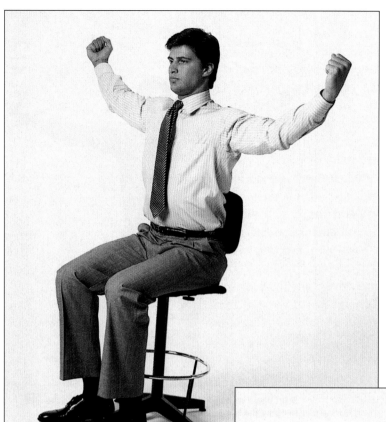

Aerobics/3

Bend your arms and extend them out to the sides, with your hands curled into fists at about ear level *(above)*. Pull your forearms towards your head *(right)*. All your movement is in the forearms; the upper arms remain stationary.

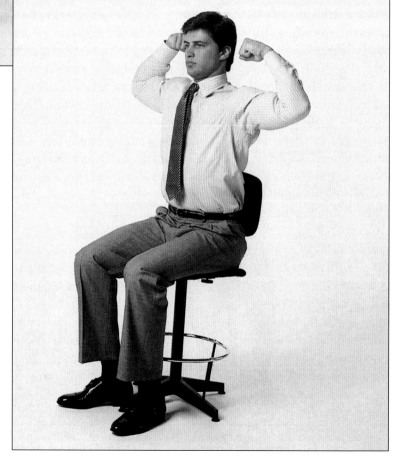

With your arms bent in front of you, move your forearms back and forth, bringing your fists towards your shoulders.

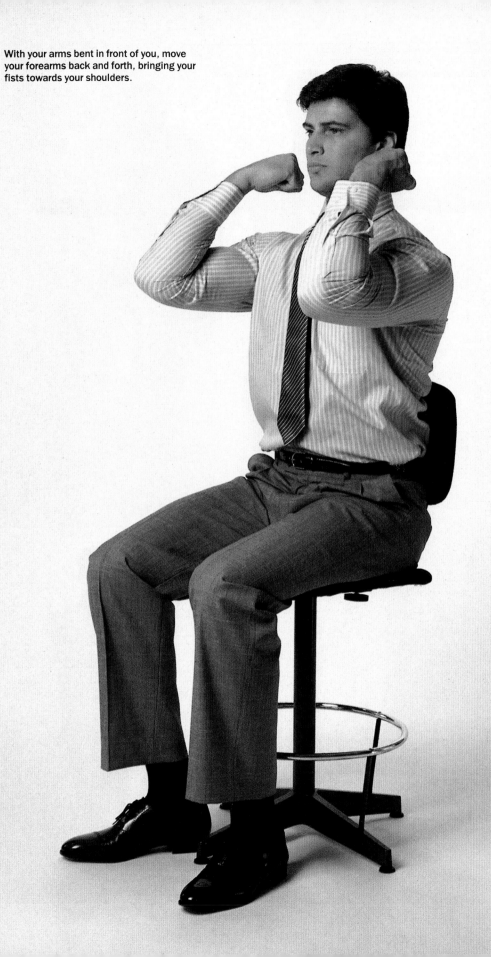

81

Aerobics/4

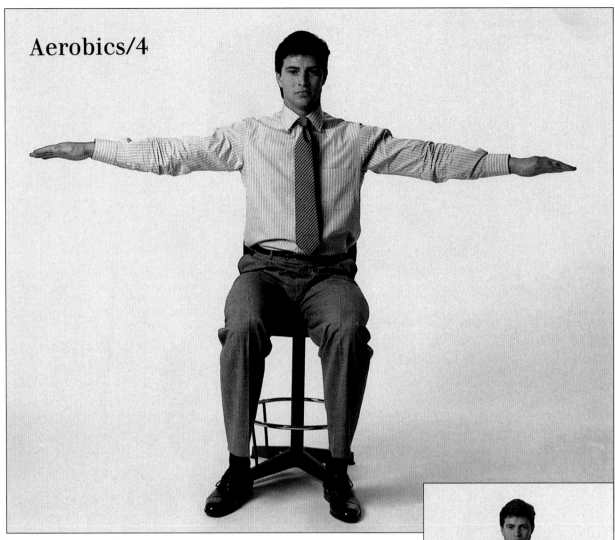

Stretch your arms open wide, palms facing down *(above)*. Swing your arms in and out, crossing them over each other when they meet at chest level. As your arms cross in front of you, lift one leg *(right)*. Repeat, alternating legs when your hands cross.

Continue crossing your arms and lifting your legs, as shown opposite. Gradually lift your arms until your hands cross above your head. For a variation, alternate flexing and pointing your toes.

Extend your right arm to the right side; bend your left arm in front of you. Form loose fists with your hands. Swing your arms together from side to side. Raise each knee alternately as your arms shift.

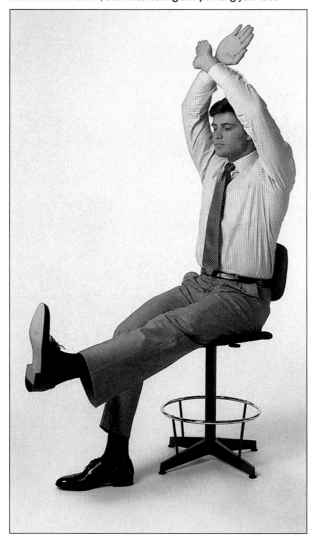
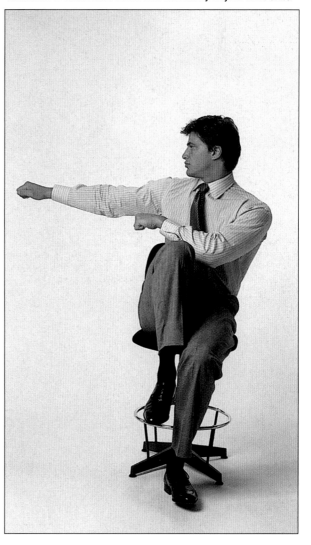

Aerobics/5

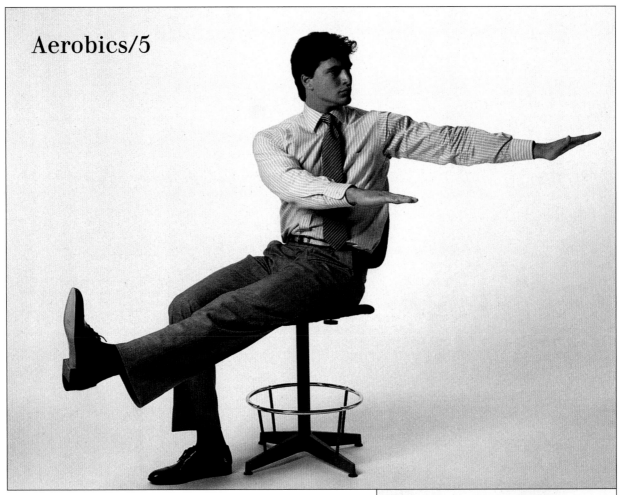

Release your fists and continue reaching to the sides in a sweeping motion, as shown on the previous page. Extend and raise your left leg, straightening your knee as you swing your arms to the left *(above)*, then your right leg as you swing your arms to the right *(right)*, alternately flexing and pointing your toes.

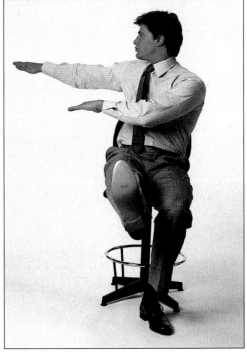

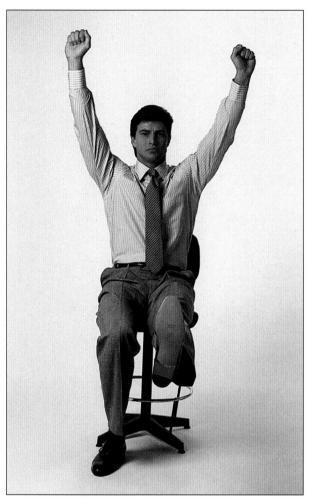

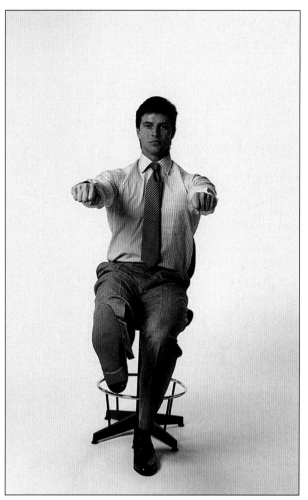

Re-forming your fists, move both hands in unison up and down as though you were lifting weights at the same time as you are lifting alternate legs.

Starting with your arms extended at shoulder level, swing them together in front of you and back, while still lifting alternate legs. To make it harder, lift your knee as you raise your leg.

Cool-Down

To cool down after completing your aerobic workout, start with shoulder shrugs, lifting each shoulder as high as you can towards your ear *(right)*. Let your hands hang down with your fingers relaxed. If you feel any tension in your hands, shake them gently. After five shoulder shrugs on each side, do 10 shrugs with both shoulders *(below)*.

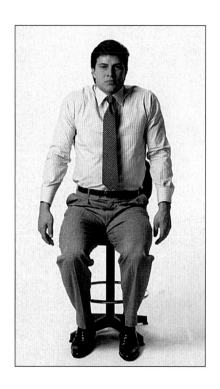

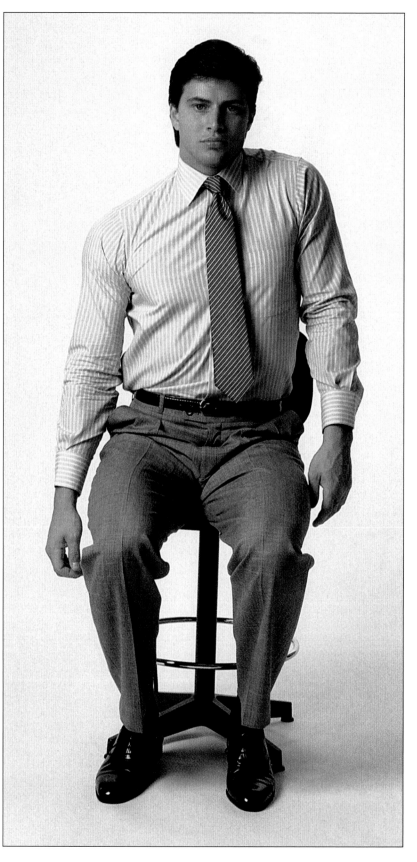

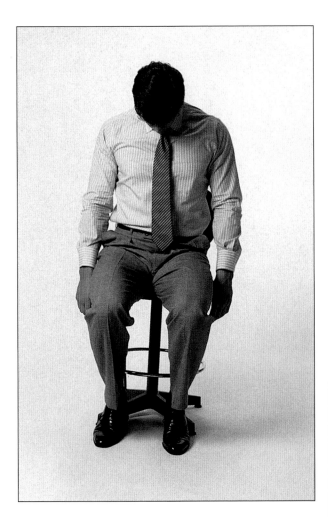

Let your chin drop to your chest and concentrate on breathing slowly, evenly and deeply. As you lift your head from this position, imagine that you are raising your neck vertebra by vertebra.

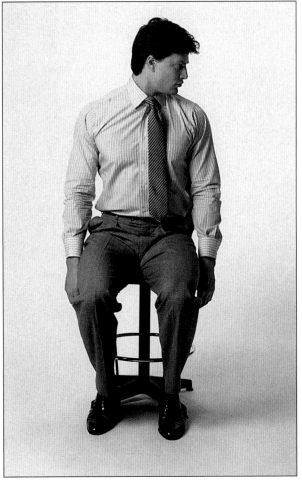

To finish the workout, turn your head slowly from side to side but avoid tilting your head backwards. Turn your head to each side as far as you can without straining your neck.

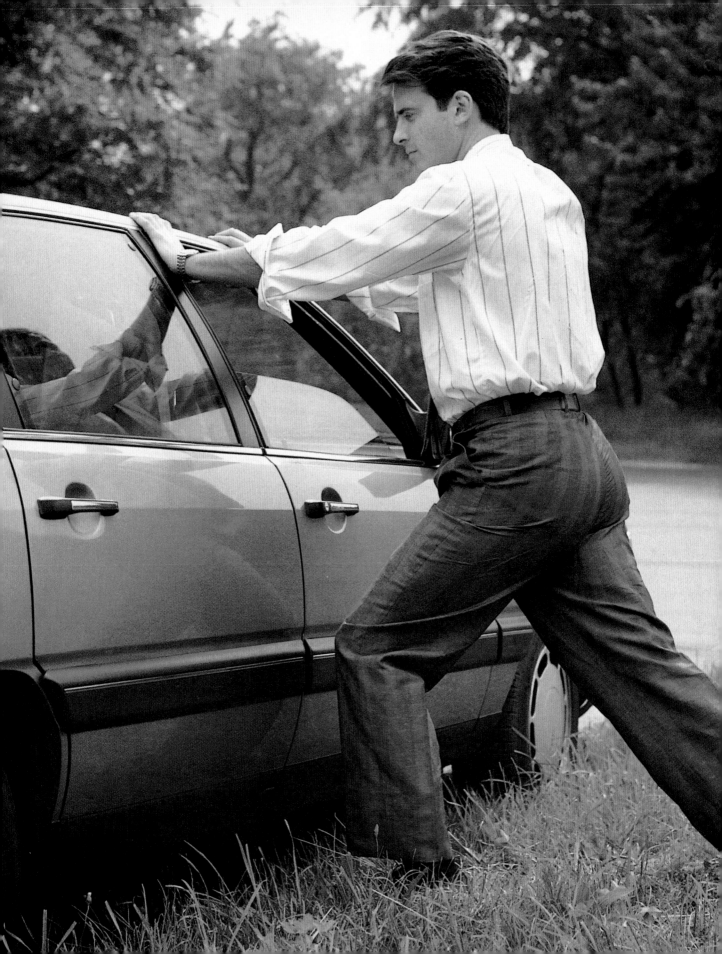

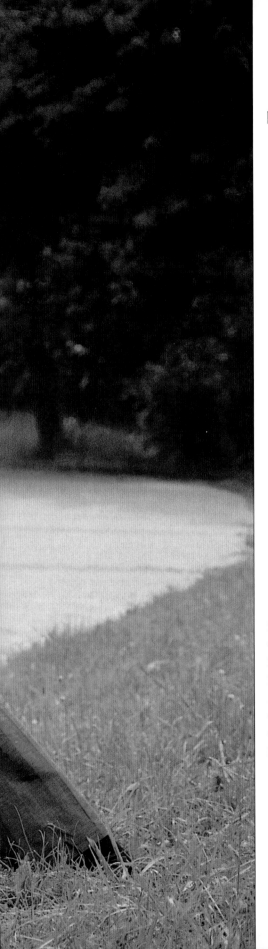

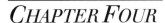
Travel Workouts

The effect of different climates and time zones on exercise, the best time for a workout, strengthening and stretching routines for confined spaces

U nless you prepare in advance, it is difficult to stay in shape while travelling. Disruptions in your every-day routine, the stress of unexpected delays, eating meals in haste or at irregular intervals, and the lack of adequate exercise facilities on the road can all interfere with a consistent fitness programme when you go away on holiday or business. While planning ahead cannot entirely counteract the negative effects of travel on your exercise regimen, it can mitigate them and save you from abandoning your commitment to fitness while you are away from home.

When you make travel plans, ask about the fitness facilities at the hotels in the area you will be visiting. Many hotels have exercise clubs and spas on the premises, and some even offer aerobics classes. Try to choose accommodation that either offers such services or allows you access to a local health club.

Be prepared, and include exercise clothing and lightweight, portable equipment such as a skipping rope when you pack for your trip. If you run, take running shoes and exercise clothing appropriate for the climate you will be visiting. If the hotel you will be staying at has a pool, take a swimming costume and goggles.

When you arrive at your destination, try to work out first thing in the morning, before you become involved in business meetings or other activities. An early workout will help you establish a fitness schedule you can follow while you are on the move. It will also help you acclimatize to any changes in time zones, counteract any stress that may have accumulated during the travel period and contribute to restful sleep at the end of the day.

As a general rule, you should not exercise as intensively when you are travelling as you do at home. You should aim for maintaining, rather than improving, fitness. Otherwise, your workouts, added to the stresses of travel, may prove too taxing, making injury or illness more likely. While you are travelling, cut your routine back to about two thirds of what you are used to and, when you return home, gradually build back up to your normal level. For instance, if you are used to running for 30 minutes a day, run for the same length of time but at a slower pace while you are away. If you need advice on where to run, a local running club may be able to provide maps with recommended routes of varying lengths.

While planning exercise in an unfamiliar place, you should also take the area's climate and altitude into account. At altitudes above 1,500 metres, for example, the air is so thin that you may experience nausea, loss of appetite, dehydration and headaches. Do not exercise as soon as you arrive when visiting high altitudes; give your body at least a day to get used to the decreased air pressure. If you usually exercise at or near sea level, you should also cut back on the duration and intensity of your exercise. The decreased atmospheric pressure at high altitudes also causes your sweat to evaporate faster, increasing your chances of becoming dehydrated. Therefore, you should drink plenty of fluids; make an effort to eat a high-carbohydrate diet with plenty of fruit and vegetables, which will help you retain fluids. If you experience an unusually rapid heartbeat or difficulty in breathing while working out in high altitudes, you should stop exercising immediately. These are both indications that your body is having trouble coping with the thin air. Finally, do not forget that being at a high altitude will affect you indoors as well as out.

You should also take similar precautions while visiting climates that are hotter than your own. In order to prevent dehydration, drink more fluids than usual, moderate your consumption of both alcohol and caffeine, which have a dehydrating effect, and try not to exercise outdoors during the hottest part of the day. To avoid sunburn, apply a sunscreen and wear a hat.

In big cities, you should forego exercising outside during morning and evening rush hours, when air pollution reaches its daily peak. If swimming is your preferred exercise, remember that swimming in the

Coping with Jet Lag

When you fly from one time zone to another, your body may become disorientated, since it has to shift its internal rhythms. Until your body adjusts to its new surroundings, you may suffer from jet lag, a condition that may be characterized by insomnia, fatigue, diarrhoea and loss of appetite. The more time zones you cross, the worse you may feel. There are several techniques you can use to alleviate the effects of jet lag:

◆ Get at least your normal amount of sleep or more every night for the week prior to departure. Three or four days before your trip, start adjusting to the time zone of your destination by shifting the timing of your daily activities. If you will be flying east, wake up and go to bed a little earlier each day; if you will be travelling west, reverse the pattern. Change your mealtimes accordingly. Make these adjustments gradually, shifting your schedule less than an hour each day.

◆ As soon as you board a plane, set your watch to the time zone you will be visiting. During the flight, you should try to sleep and eat as though you were in the new time zone. When you reach your destination, avoid taking a nap immediately. If possible, participate in normal business and social activities, and spend time outdoors. Researchers believe that exposure to daylight stimulates the release of hormones that help co-ordinate your internal bodily rhythms with the local time.

◆ Schedule important meetings or long drives for a time when you would be awake at home. Jet lag can affect your mental acuity, lowering your ability to concentrate and impairing your memory and performance. It can also slow your reflexes. Some studies have shown that these detrimental effects are especially strong when you are awake in a new time zone but would usually be asleep at home.

sea can be dangerous for those who usually swim in a calm lake or pool — strong swimmers included. Do not swim alone or at beaches where there are no lifeguards.

The time that elapses between leaving home and reaching your destination can add significantly to the stress of travel. Standing in long queues at terminals or sitting in the same position for hours on planes, buses, trains or in cars can cause muscle cramps, fatigue and feelings of malaise. The best antidote to the confinement of long trips is to get up periodically and walk about. Walking works the large muscles in your legs and restores circulation to your extremities. In tight spaces such as the cabin of a crowded plane, where walking about frequently may not be possible, the exercises that are presented in this chapter will be especially beneficial. The movements include stretches, isometrics and other exercises that you can perform almost anywhere — even while you are standing in a queue.

Regardless of your mode of transport, the exercises will offset the boredom and help to counteract the debilitating effects of long trips. As a result, they will make you feel better when you reach your destination than you would have if you had simply sat still.

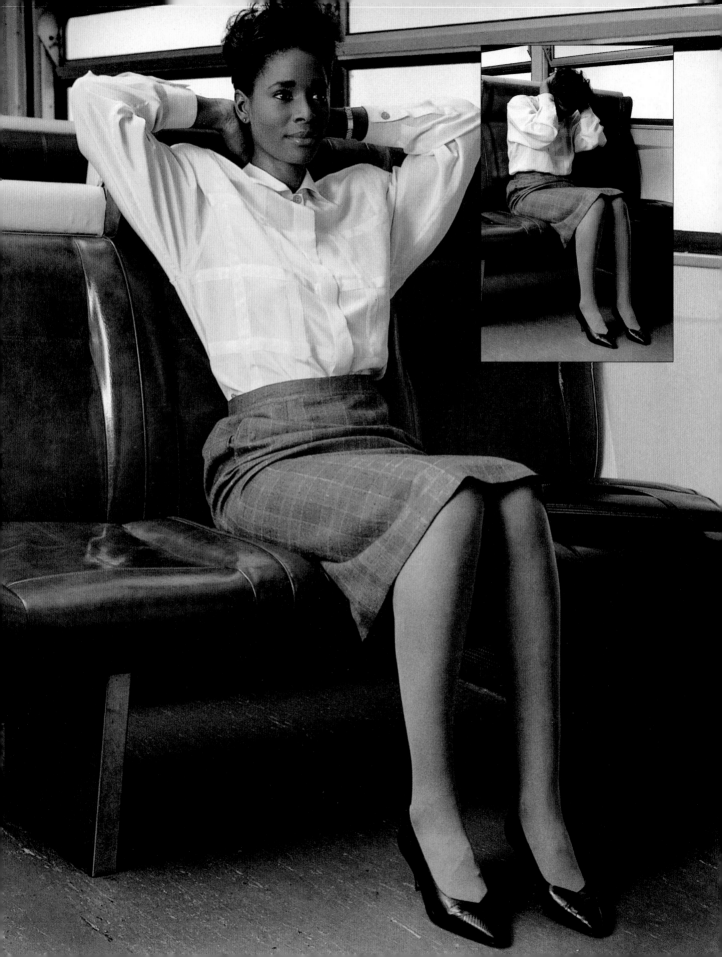

Stretches

Cramps, stiffness and numbness can be problems for travellers who are confined to their seats during long rides in cars, buses, trains or aeroplanes. Car and bus travellers, whose muscles may be subjected to jarring motions in stop-and-go traffic, are especially vulnerable to muscle spasms, particularly in the back. But exercises that involve gentle stretching will alleviate such discomforts. If possible, sit in an aisle seat, as this will give you more room in which to perform these movements.

If you do not stretch and move around as you travel, you run the risk of suffering undue fatigue when you reach your destination. And stiff, cramped muscles can make it uncomfortable to resume normal movement on arrival. So if your schedule or travel arrangements prevent you from performing any other type of exercise while you are away from home, you should at least do the loosening and flexibility-enhancing routines shown on these and the following two pages. You can begin performing them when you are en route to your destination and continue doing them at least once a day, and more if you wish, upon arrival.

A technique that increases the effectiveness of stretching is to contract the muscles you are about to stretch for a moment and then, as you stretch, consciously relax them. The brief contraction stimulates a reflex that helps to lengthen the muscles. Consciously relaxing them increases your awareness of the tension that builds up in these parts of the body, so try not to let your mind wander as you stretch.

The stretches focus on the areas that tend to tighten the most when you are travelling — the muscles of the neck, shoulders and lower back. When you perform the stretches shown here, the movement should be relaxed: do not force your joints beyond a comfortable range of motion. Above all, do not stretch so far as to cause pain.

You should keep your muscles loose and relaxed as you do the movement exercises shown on pages 94-97. Avoid exaggerated movements and do not stretch any farther than feels comfortable. Hold each stretch for 30 to 45 seconds.

Sit up straight and interlace your fingers behind your head, pointing your elbows out to the sides *(opposite)*. Bring your elbows towards each other and press gently with your hands until your chin reaches your chest *(inset)*. Hold.

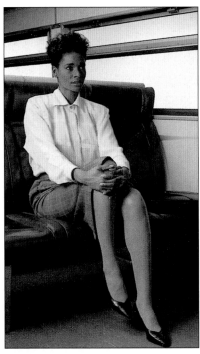

Place your hands over one knee. Pull your leg up until you feel a slight stretch in your thigh. Hold. Repeat with the other leg.

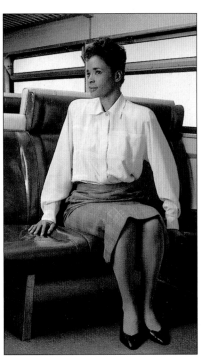

Turn to one side, rotating from the waist, until you feel a stretch in your lower back. Hold. Repeat on the other side.

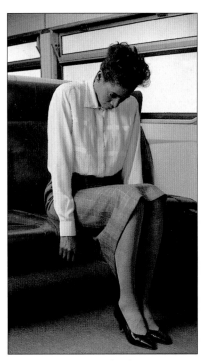

Sit with your arms hanging loosely at your sides. Gently let your chin fall to your chest. Hold this position.

Shoulder Stretches

Look straight ahead and cross your arms in your lap, keeping your shoulders relaxed *(right)*. Slowly bring your arms up in front of you *(far right and below, left)*. Lift your hands above your head *(below, centre)* and bring them up and out to the sides. Making as large a circle as possible with your hands and arms *(below, right)*, slowly bring them back to the starting position. Do five repetitions.

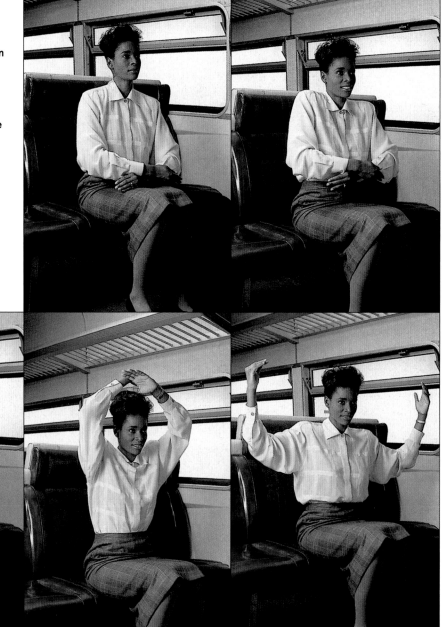

Extend your arms and grasp the bottom of your seat. Keeping your back as straight as possible, pull up firmly on the seat without straining *(opposite)*. As you pull, lean back until you feel a slight stretch in your shoulders. Hold.

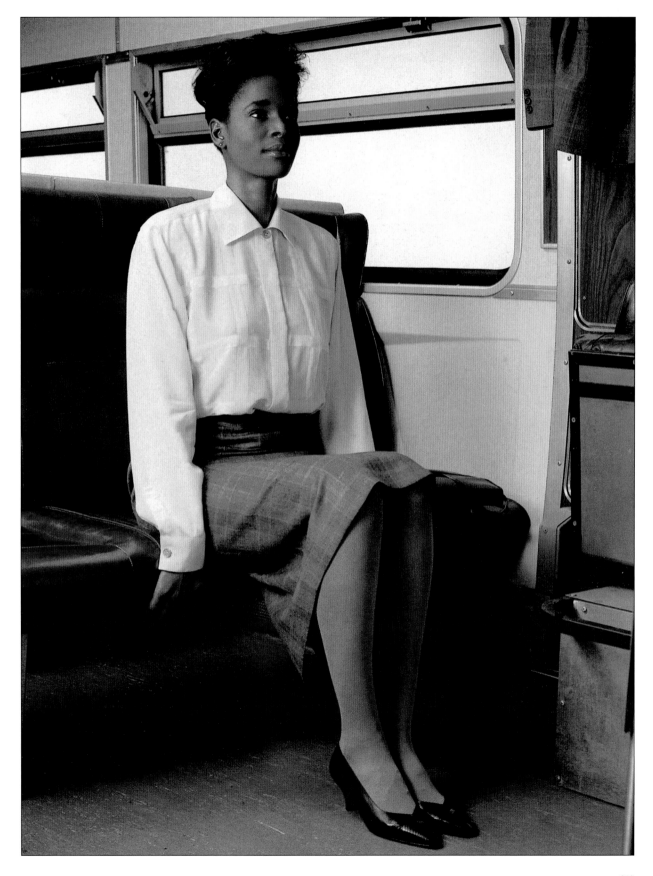

Chest Stretches

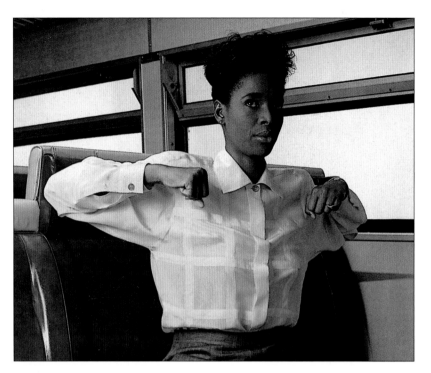

Curl your hands into fists and hold them in front of your chest, your elbows out to the sides. Reach back with your elbows *(left)* until you feel a stretch across the middle of your chest and upper chest. Hold. As you move your elbows back, you may have to lean forwards slightly to have enough room to complete the stretch.

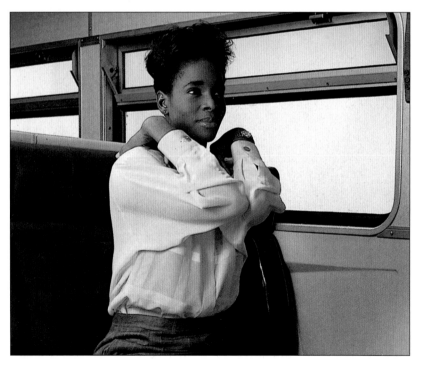

Place your hands on your shoulders. Bring your elbows together in front of you as your shoulder blades move apart *(left)*. Hold.

Press your hands together in front of you, the fingers pointing up *(opposite)*. Look straight ahead. As you continue gently pressing your hands together, lift them over your head as high as you can *(inset)*. Then slowly lower them to the starting position. Do five repetitions.

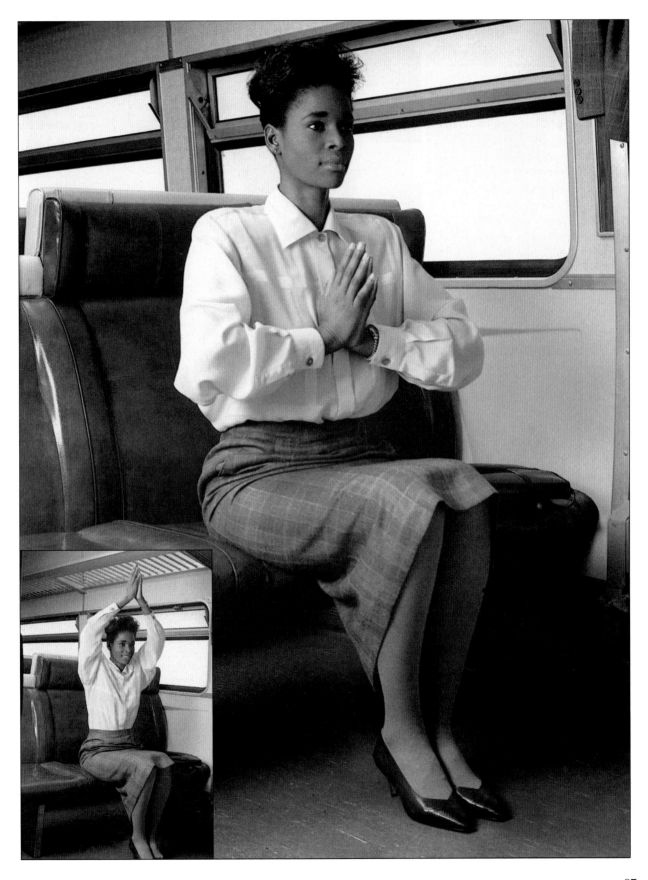

Strength Builders

In a crowded passenger compartment, strengthening exercises are the most inconspicuous ones that you can perform. They generally require a minimum of space and do not interfere with other travellers. Isometrics, which involve static muscle contractions and entail no movement once you have assumed the proper position, need less space than dynamic exercises, or isotonics, which do require some degree of movement.

Nearly all the isometrics shown on pages 98-103 oppose one body part with another. You can perform these on virtually any kind of chair and in any vehicle. The two exceptions — which require a large high-backed chair or padded seat — are the backwards push against the seat (*page 99*) and the push downwards on the cushion (*page 101*). You will probably not be able to perform either of these exercises in a very crowded space, or sitting in a chair with a very narrow seat or back.

As you perform the isometrics, remember to do each one at several different angles, since isometrics develop strength only at the particular angle at which they are performed. For each isometric exercise, push as hard as you can for about 10 seconds and continue to breathe evenly.

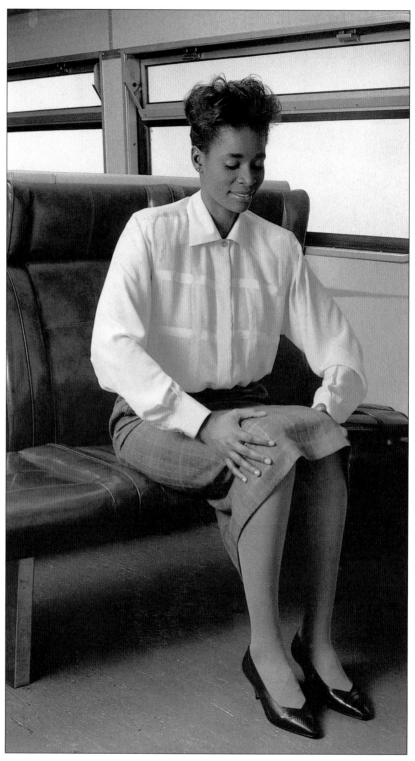

Sit with your knees about 15 centimetres apart. Press your hands against the outside of your knees. Push outwards with your thigh muscles so that you resist the hand pressure. The farther you extend your elbows, the more you work your chest.

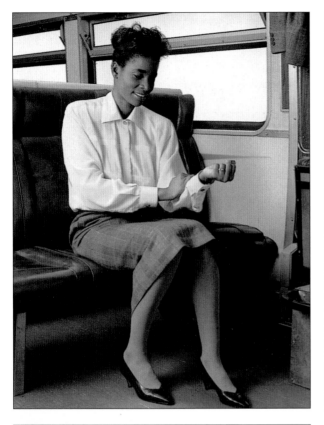

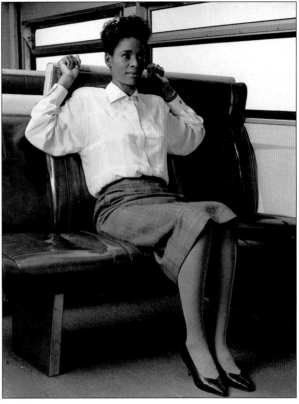

Hold your left arm out, bent at the elbow, palm up. Push down on the arm with the right hand and resist with the left arm *(above, left)*. Lean back in your seat. Bend your arms so that your elbows extend to the side and your hands rest on the top of the seat. Press your hands back against the seat *(above)*. Sit up straight with one palm resting on your forehead. Press against your forehead and resist with your neck muscles *(left)*.

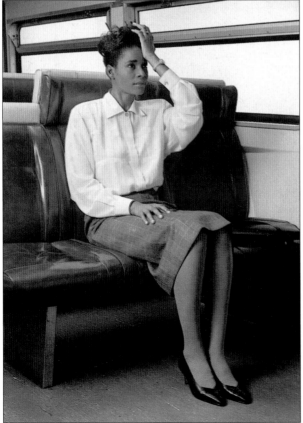

Arm Isometrics/1

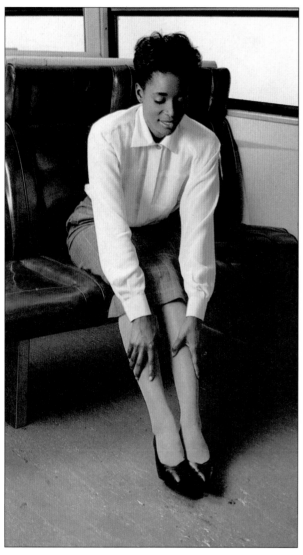

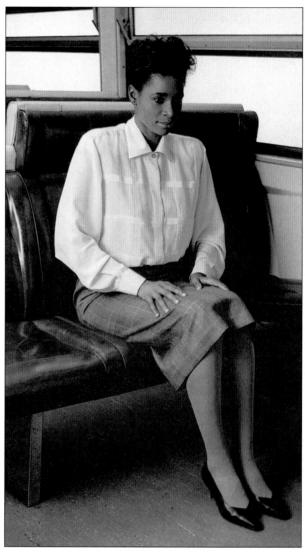

Lean forwards and place your hands on your shins. Keep your back straight and push against your legs.

Place your hands on top of your thighs and press down. To work your thigh muscles, resist by trying to lift your legs.

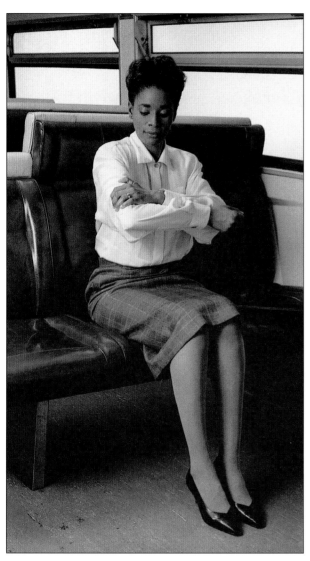

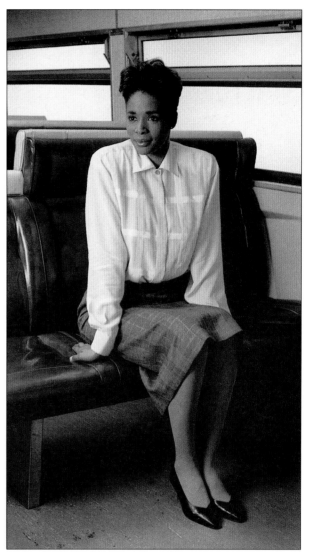

Fold your arms. Grasp your right upper arm with your left hand and pull as your right arm resists. Repeat on the other side.

Put your hands on your seat, fingers pointing behind you. Keep your arms straight and push down on the seat.

Arm Isometrics/2

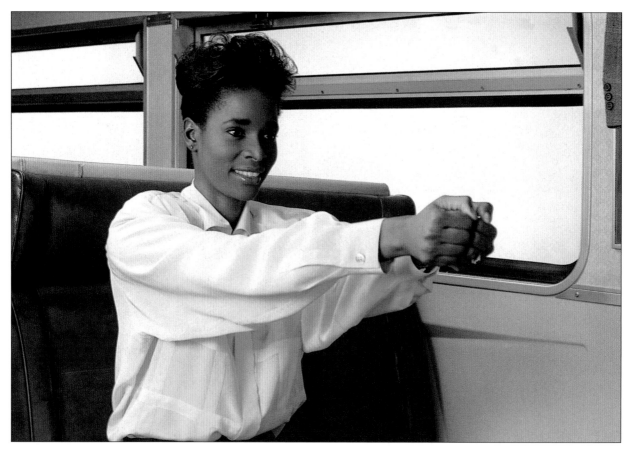

Hold your arms straight out in front of you.
Make two fists and hold them together with
knuckles touching. Push your arms
together. To vary the angle, move your fists
slowly towards your chest and then away
from you as you press them together.

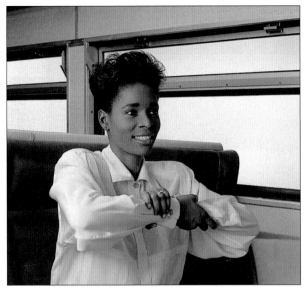

Cross your arms and grasp each forearm with the opposite hand. Pull outwards and then push the other way.

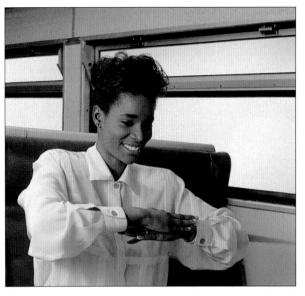

Put one hand on top of the other in front of you. Push your hands against each other, then switch hands.

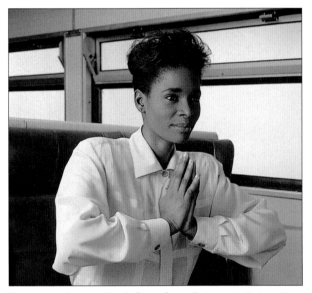

Place your palms together in front of you, fingers pointing up. Press your hands together.

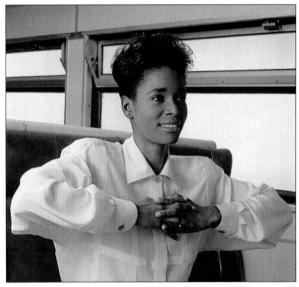

Interlock your fingers in front of your chest and pull outwards. Reverse directions and push your hands towards each other.

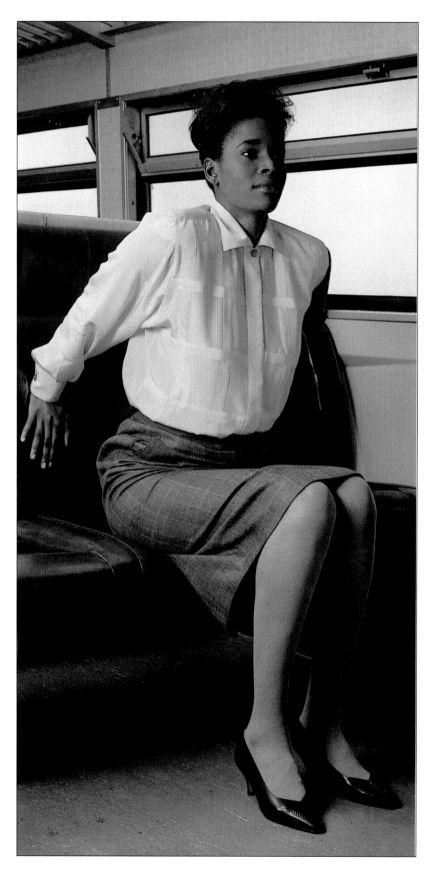

Arm Strengtheners

Lean forwards and press your hands against the back of the seat, keeping your arms straight and your fingers pointing down. Keep your back as straight as possible and push against the seat. Repeat several times, varying the distance between your hands.

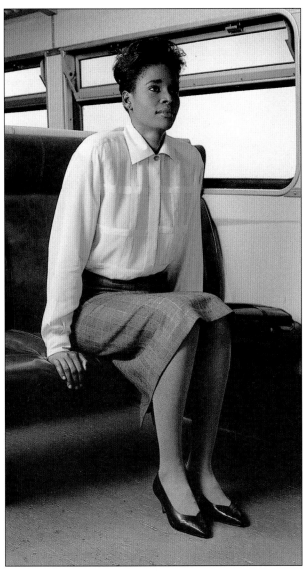

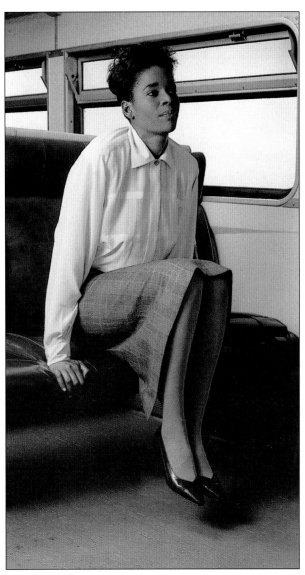

Sitting up straight, grasp the edge of your seat with your hands. First push down as hard as you can and hold, then pull up and hold.

Grip the edge of the seat with both hands; lift and lower yourself three times. Do not do this if you have lower back problems.

Leg and Stomach Strengtheners

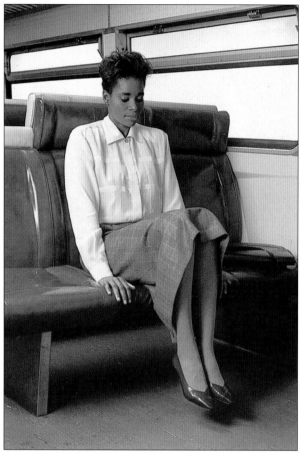

Rest your palms against your seat. Lift your knees towards your chest and then slowly lower them. Do five repetitions.

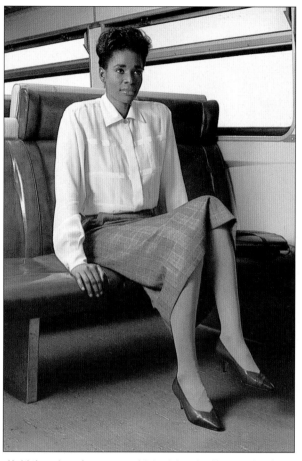

Hold the edge of your seat with both hands. Alternately raise and lower each knee 15 centimetres. Do 20 repetitions.

With both feet on the floor, first lift the heel *(opposite)* and then the toe *(inset)* of each foot in a rocking motion. Do 10 repetitions with each foot.

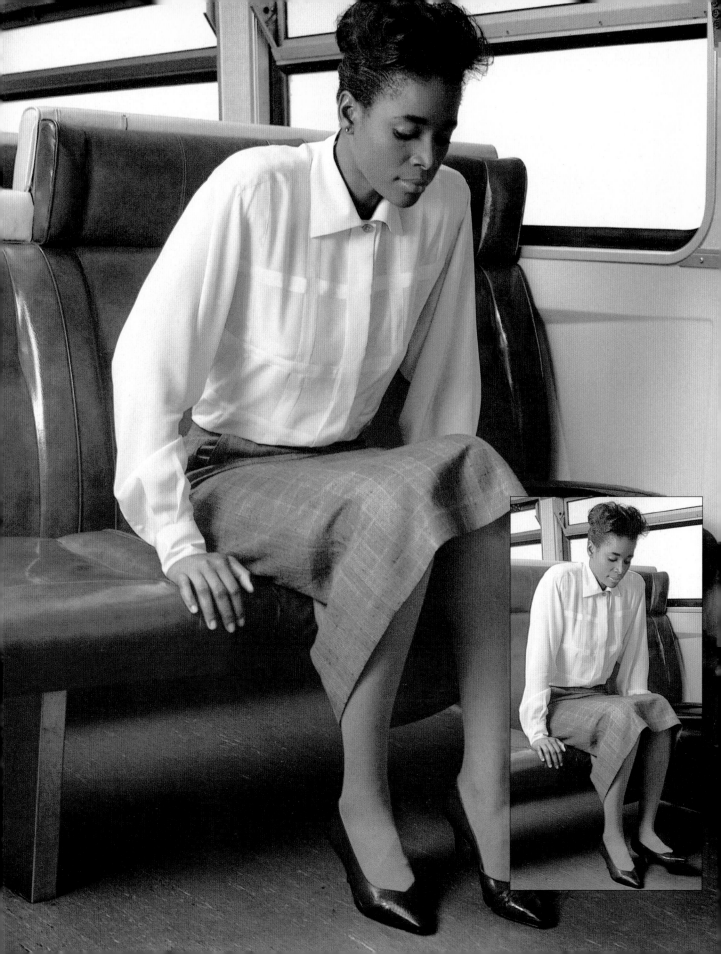

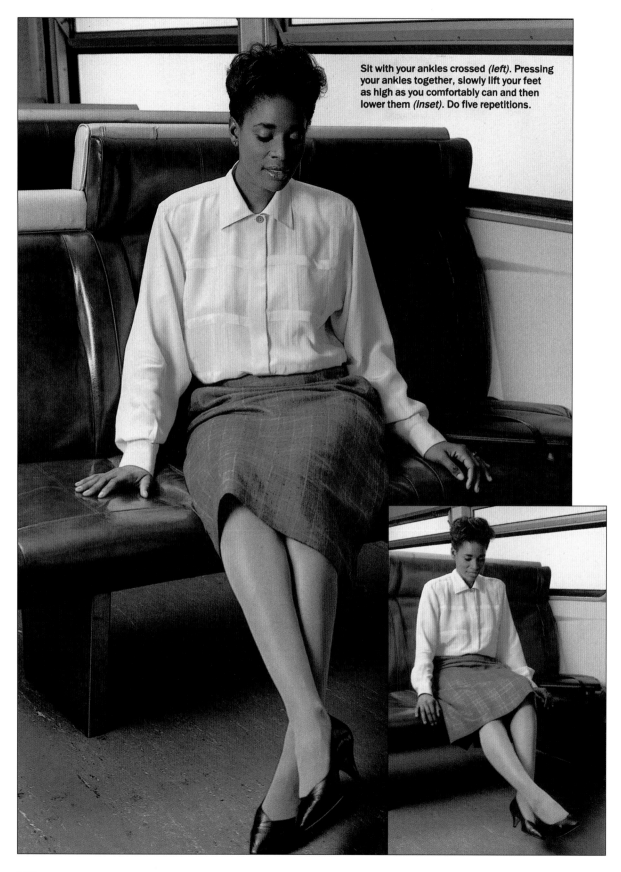

Sit with your ankles crossed *(left)*. Pressing your ankles together, slowly lift your feet as high as you comfortably can and then lower them *(inset)*. Do five repetitions.

Leg Strengtheners

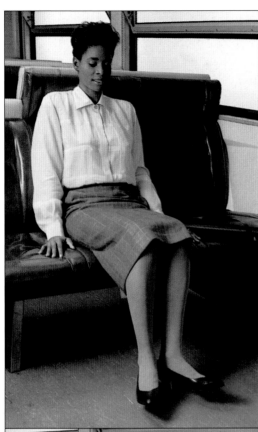

Push your ankles together as you point your toes out at a 45-degree angle *(left)*. Hold your legs out straight and push your feet together *(below, left)*. Sit with your legs straight or knees slightly bent and flex your toes. Press your heels together *(below)*.

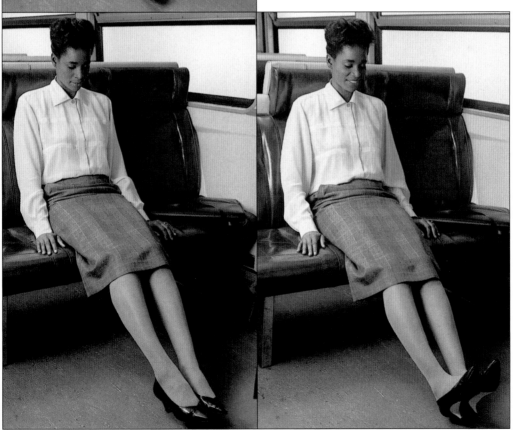

Travel Posture

The way you sit on a long trip will affect the way you feel when you reach your destination. While stretches and other exercises are important in preventing cramps, stiffness and muscular tension, maintaining proper posture is also necessary for preventing these discomforts from developing into serious problems.

When sitting, avoid crossing your legs at the knees, which pulls on the lower back and can strain it. Such a position also stresses the knees and can restrict blood circulation to your lower legs.

One of the best ways to sit is to keep both of your feet flat on the floor. Two other recommended positions, shown on the opposite page, are crossing one ankle over a knee and crossing your ankles.

When you are reading, lift your book or magazine and keep your neck and shoulders upright, as shown in the photograph on the right below. If you hold your book in your lap and have to bend to read it, you can strain your neck, shoulders and upper back as you hunch over.

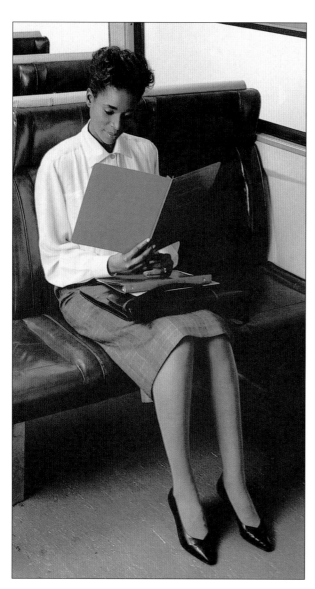

Whenever possible, put a bag or briefcase on your lap to support your arms while you hold a book or magazine.

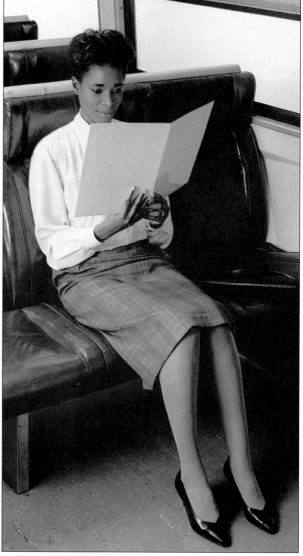

Never hunch over while reading when you travel. Bring your work or reading matter up towards your face.

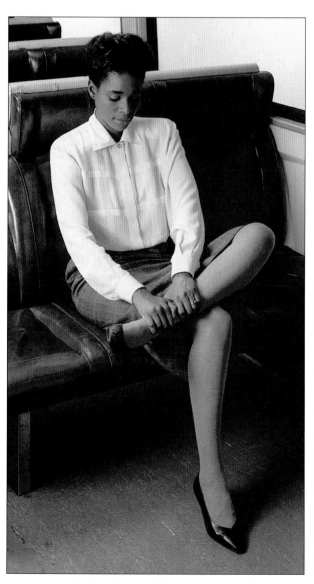

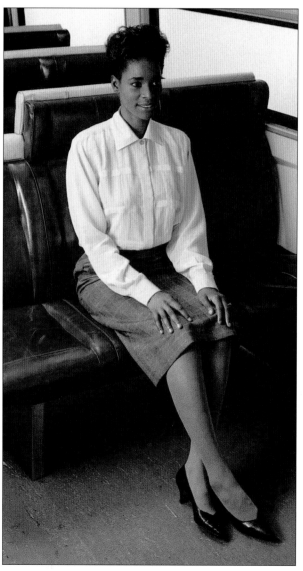

Do not cross your knees when sitting. Crossing an ankle over one knee is better for your lower back.

Crossing your ankles or sitting with your feet together and flat on the floor is the best sitting posture.

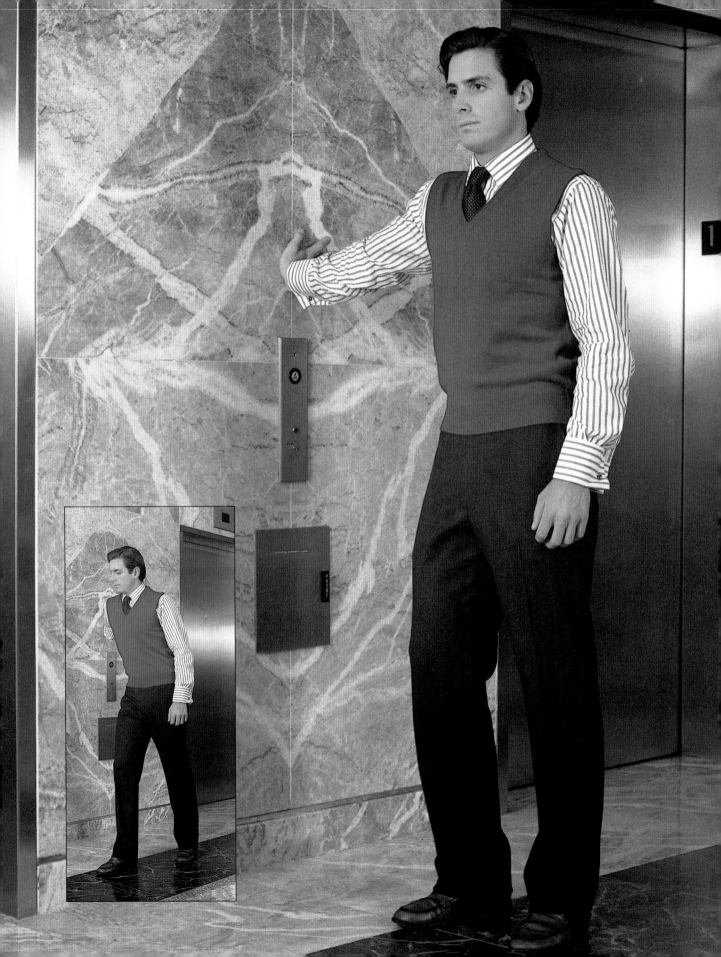

Standing Stretches

When standing in a queue or waiting for a lift, keep moving. Do not hold the same position for an extended period. Move your hands, step back and forth, stretch, take off your jacket or coat, put down your bag and pick it up, and devise other stratagems to keep yourself from standing still. The motion of your arm and leg muscles will aid your circulation and keep blood from pooling in the veins in your legs.

Curiously, standing still can be more stressful than moving about. For example, standing in one place with your knees locked and your legs straight places too much of the burden of support for your body on your back. It is better to stand with one leg slightly extended in front of the other and your knees bent. By doing this, you place demands on the muscles in your thighs, abdomen and hips, but not your back.

Waiting for a lift in any uncrowded place gives you the chance to perform the stretches shown on these two pages. The stretch shown on the opposite page is good for relieving the tension and stiffness that carrying a heavy briefcase or handbag for a long time can produce in your shoulders. The lunge shown on this page stretches the muscles in the lower legs. Hold each stretch for 30 to 45 seconds.

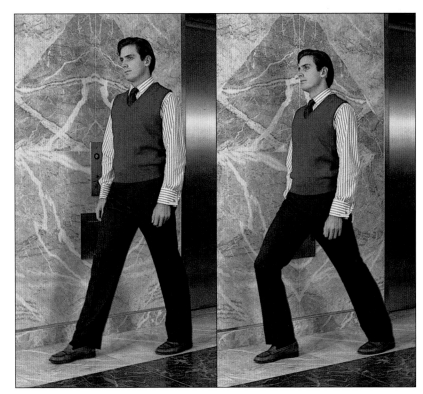

Stand with your right foot about 30 centimetres in front of the left. Let your arms hang loosely at your sides *(above)*. Lunge forwards gently, bending your knees so that you lower your upper body about 15 centimetres *(above, right)*. Keep your back straight. Hold. Reverse feet and repeat.

Stand with your right shoulder near the wall, your right foot slightly in front of the left. Reach out with your right hand and place the palm on the wall, fingers pointing to the rear *(opposite)*. Keeping your hand at the same spot on the wall, slide your right foot and shoulder forwards until you feel a stretch in your shoulder *(inset)*. Hold. Then turn round and repeat.

Lower Body Strengtheners

The wall of a waiting room or lobby is the only equipment you need to work on the muscles of your lower body. Of course, you could perform general lower body strengtheners without leaning against something, but using a wall for support better enables you to do exercises for your legs and stomach that work one side of the body at a time.

The leg lifts shown on this page and at the bottom of the opposite page work the muscles of the thigh, buttocks and, to a more limited extent, the lower stomach. Movements that involve lifting a leg out to the side develop the outer thigh muscles (*opposite, bottom right*); and movements that involve crossing the legs (*opposite, bottom left*) strengthen the inner thigh.

Exercises that bring the knees towards the chest, such as the one shown in the top two photographs opposite and the exercise shown on the right of page 117, focus mostly on the stomach muscles. Bending from the waist, as shown on page 116, also develops the back muscles.

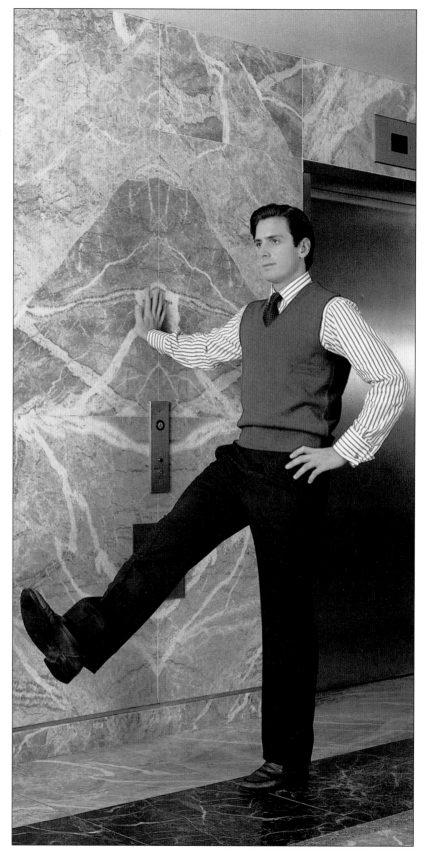

Stand up straight and place your feet together. Put your left hand on your hip and your right hand on the wall. Keeping your right leg straight, bring it forwards, lifting it as high as you can, and then lower it. Do 10 repetitions, then turn round and repeat with the other leg.

114

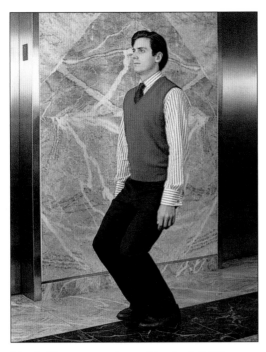

Stand with your arms at your sides, feet slightly apart. Bend your knees and lower your trunk about 15 centimetres. Keeping your back straight and your head up, rise back up to the starting position. Do five repetitions.

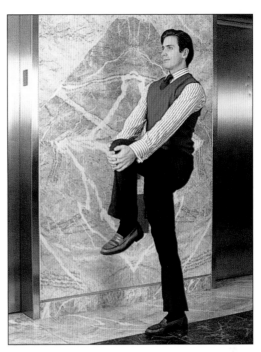

Stand with your feet together. Raise your left knee, grasp it with both hands and lift it as high as you can without straining. Hold, then switch knees. Use the wall for support if necessary.

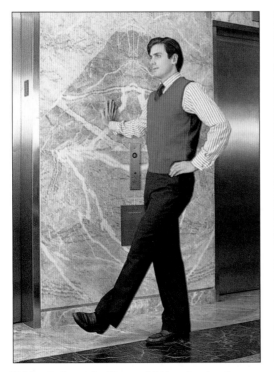

Hold on to the wall with your right hand and rest your left hand on your hip. Swing your left leg forwards, keeping it straight, and then swing it towards the wall. Bring it back next to the right leg. Do 10 repetitions. Turn round and repeat on the other side.

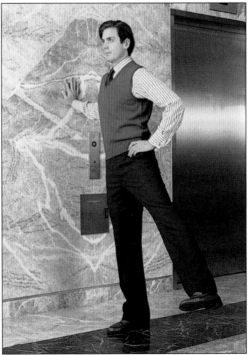

Stand with your right hand on the wall for support. Lift your left leg out to the side, keeping it straight. Bring it back down slowly until it is next to your right foot. Do five repetitions. Then turn round and repeat on the other side.

Stomach Strengtheners

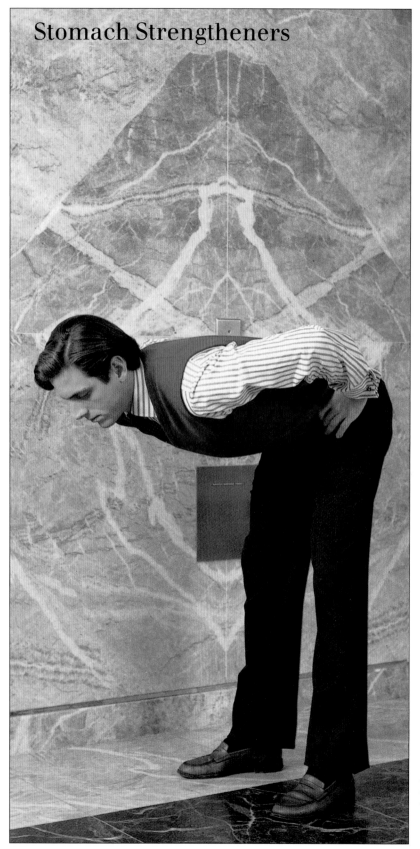

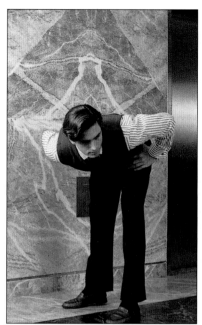

Standing with your hands on your hips, knees slightly bent, bend forwards from the waist and turn your trunk to the left. Return to the centre and stand up straight. Do five repetitions. Repeat to the other side.

Stand with your hands on your hips. Your knees should be slightly bent, not locked. Place your feet so that your toes form an angle of about 45 degrees. Bend forwards slowly from the waist as far as you comfortably can, but do not let your head drop below the level of your buttocks. Return to the starting position. Do five repetitions.

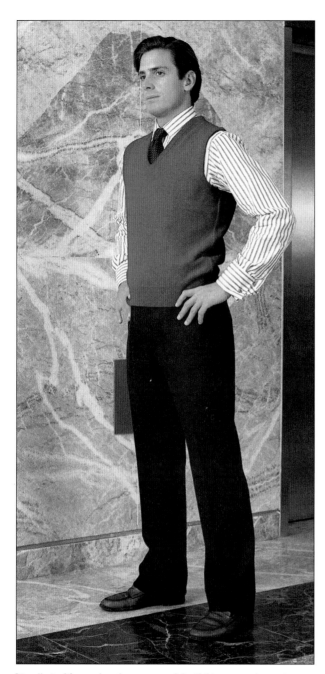

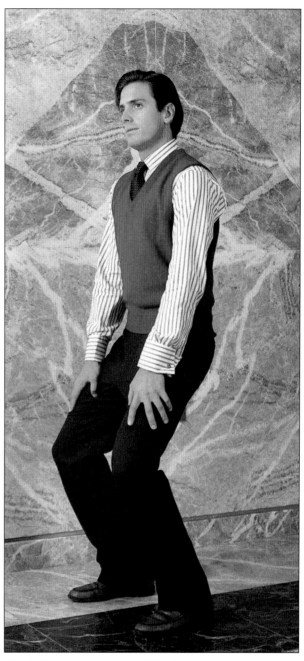

Standing with your hands on your pelvis, tighten your stomach muscles. Press your hands against your hips as you turn your trunk slightly to the left. Return to the starting position. Do five repetitions on each side.

Stand with your hands on your thighs. Tense your stomach muscles as you drop your buttocks about 15 centimetres and press on your legs with your hands, keeping your back straight. Return to the starting position. Do 10 repetitions.

One-Minute Routines

Waiting in a lobby gives you an ideal opportunity to do isometrics and dynamic strengthening that you cannot do in the confines of a crowded bus, train or plane. Pushing against a wall while standing, for example, uses most of the major muscles of the upper body. After doing these exercises, you should relax by doing one or more of the stretches shown on pages 122-123. Hold each stretch for 30 to 60 seconds.

The exercises that involve pushing against a wall can be done as isometrics when you push and then hold a steady position, or as dynamic exercises when you move slowly as you push. The isometrics should be held for approximately 10 seconds. Dynamic exercises can be done for 10 to 20 repetitions.

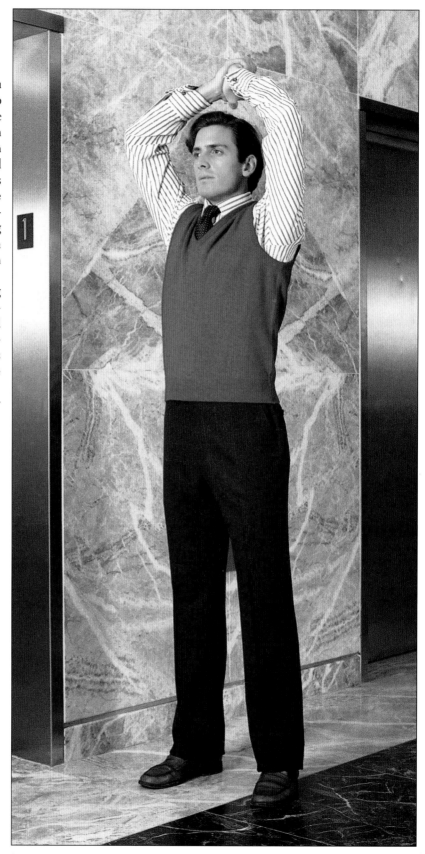

Stand with your hands together over your head. Press them against each other and hold.

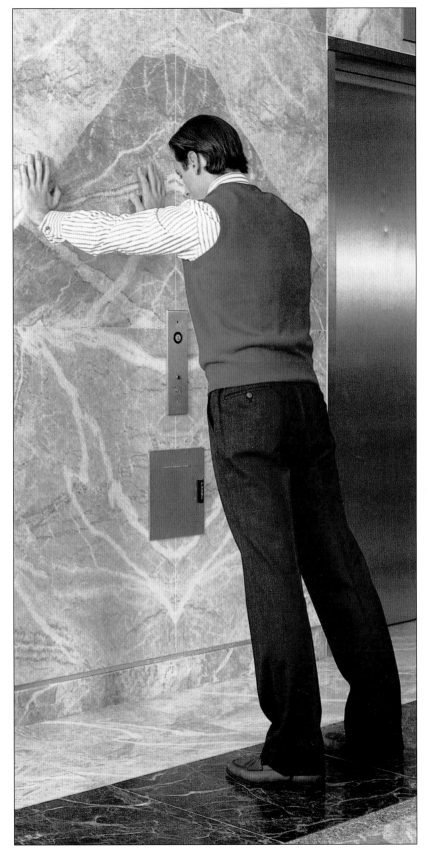

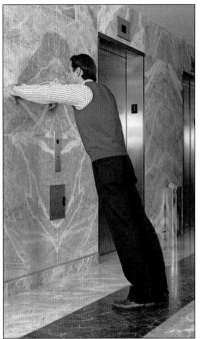

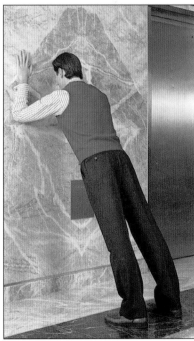

With your feet about 1 metre from a wall, place your hands on the wall at shoulder level, keeping your arms and back straight and fingers pointed up. Push *(left)*. From the same starting position, rotate your hands so that your fingers point inwards. Bend your elbows slightly and push *(top)*. Place your forearms on the wall, fingers again pointing up, and push *(above)*.

Strengtheners

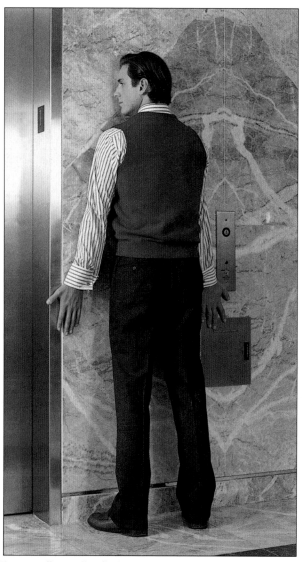

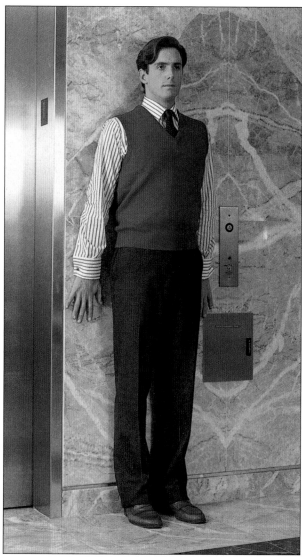

Face a wall, standing flush against it, your head turned to one side. With your arms at your sides, rest your palms against the wall, fingers pointing down. Push your hands against the wall.

Stand with your back to the wall with your arms hanging down. Keeping your arms and legs straight, place your palms against the wall and push with your hands.

Stand 30 centimetres away from a wall. Lean forwards, placing your forearms on the wall, hands pointing up. Bend your right knee and move your left foot back about 60 centimetres, keeping your left leg straight. Push as hard as you can, concentrating all the effort in your legs (opposite).

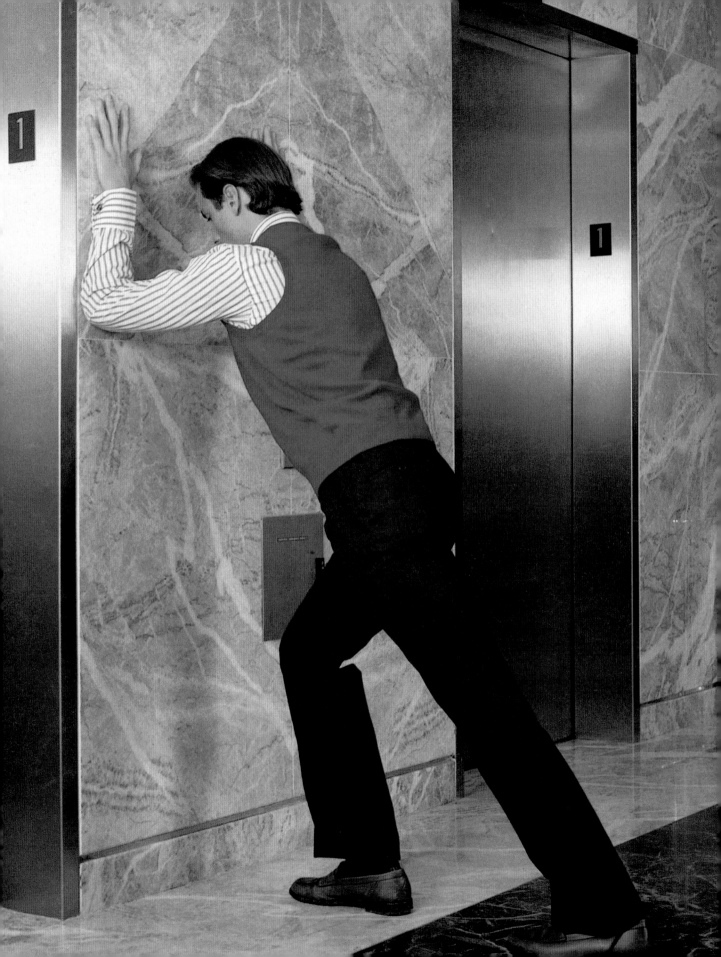

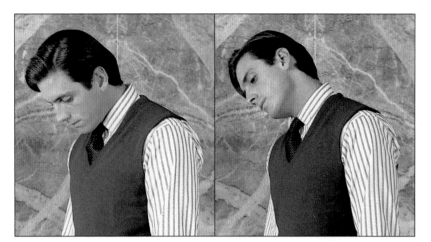

Stretches

Stand with your arms relaxed at your sides and let your chin fall to your chest *(far left)*. Rotate your head to the right until your chin is level with your shoulder *(left)*. Return to the centre position. Do five repetitions on each side.

With your knees slightly bent, gently lean forwards. Let your hands reach for the floor *(left)*, but do not force yourself down or bounce in an effort to touch the floor. Keep your knees slightly bent.

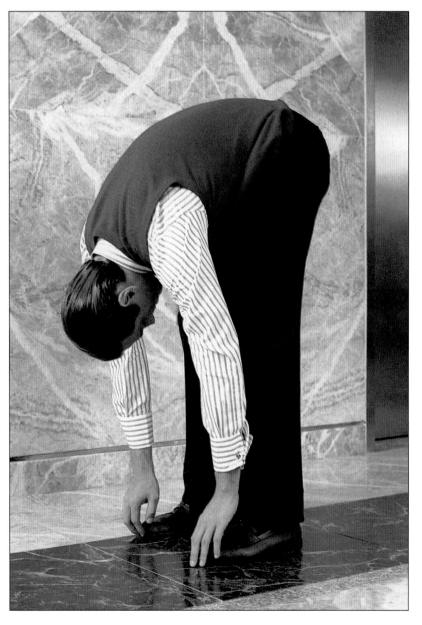

Stand up straight with your feet shoulder width apart. Reach up as high as you can and hold *(opposite)*.

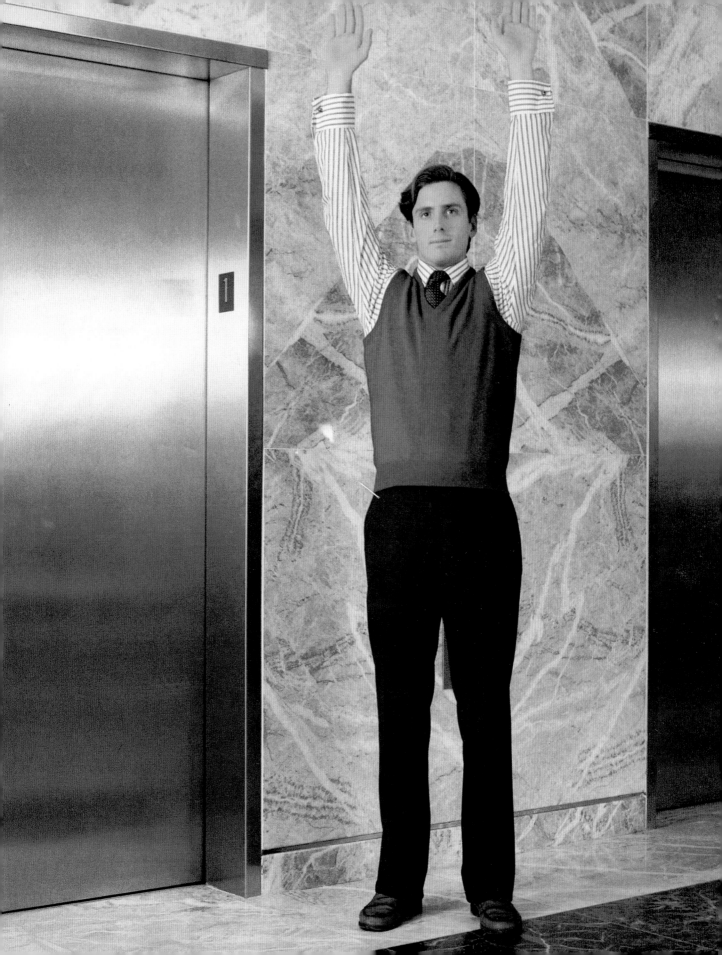

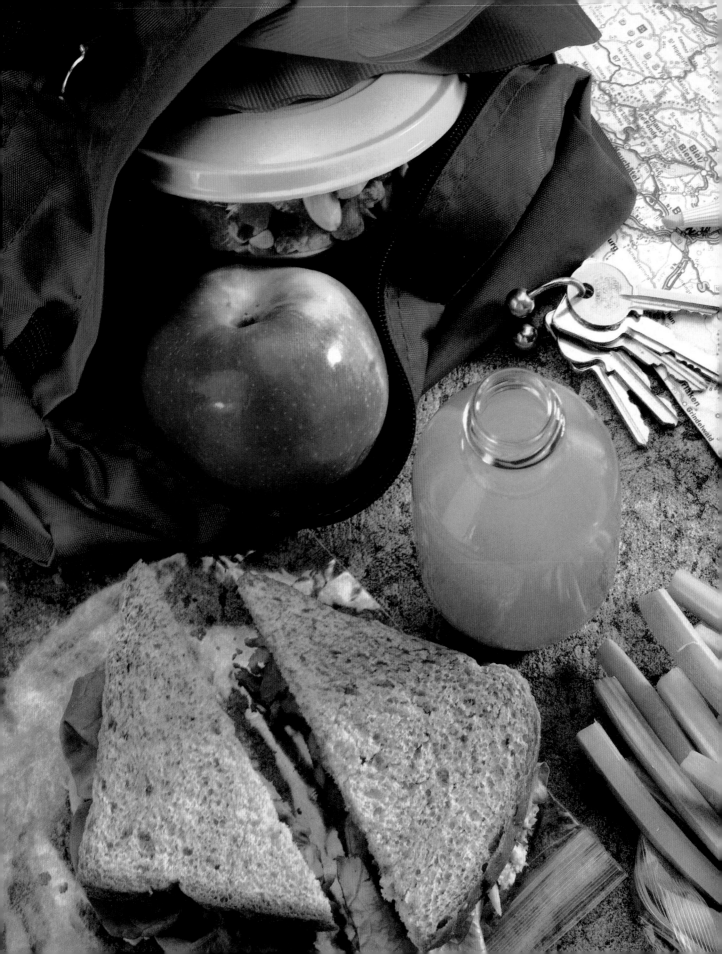

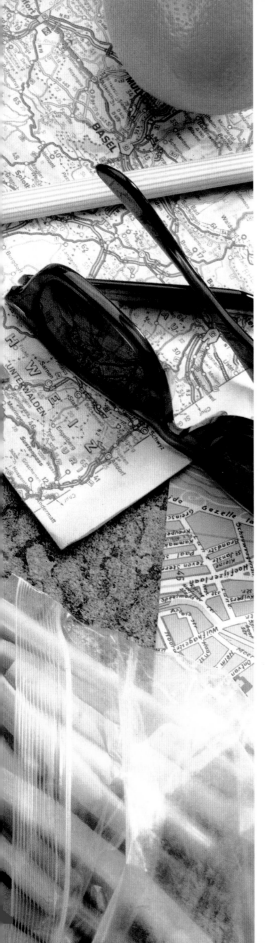

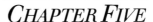
Eating on the Go

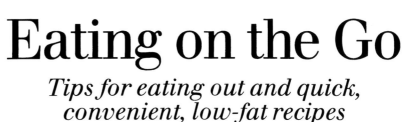

Tips for eating out and quick, convenient, low-fat recipes

Fast-food restaurants and snack bars are ubiquitous and convenient. But the food they serve reflects the trend towards unhealthy eating that, during most of this century, has characterized the modern diet — most markedly in the amount of fat and sugar that are consumed.

The fat content of most fast-food meals poses a particular risk to human health. Studies have shown that a diet high in fat, especially the saturated fat found in animal products, is associated with heart disease and various types of cancer, as well as with obesity. Yet many fast-food products derive half or more of their calories from fat. More than 50 per cent of the calories in a take-away ham and cheese sandwich come from fat. In hot dogs, up to 60 per cent of the calories come from fat. Hamburgers, too, are packed with saturated fat, and although fish and the white meat of chicken are ordinarily lower in saturated fat than beef, the fish and chicken dishes in fast-food restaurants are

125

usually fried in beef fat or coconut or palm oil, which have a higher saturated fat content than butter. Because fat has more than twice as many calories by weight as protein or carbohydrates, frying foods can substantially increase their caloric content. For example, a plain 250-gram baked potato, which is high in complex carbohydrates, contains 250 calories; by contrast, just half the quantity of French fries contains 350 calories — a substantial proportion of a day's calorie intake.

This chapter offers recipes that provide low-fat alternatives that are easy to make and convenient to carry. For example, the Double Potato Salad on page 135 derives only 4 per cent of its calories from fat, as compared with conventional potato salad, which is more than 50 per cent fat. The reason for the reduction in fat is simple: rather than relying on mayonnaise, a snack-bar staple that is nearly 100 per cent fat, this recipe uses low-fat buttermilk-and-yogurt dressing. Similarly, the Cinnamon-Peachy Shake *(page 141)* is made with low-fat vanilla yogurt instead of whole milk and ice cream — and this gives it about one third the fat content of a typical fast-food shake.

In addition to their excess fat, many fast foods are loaded with sodium in the form of salt — and, in susceptible individuals, consuming too much sodium has been associated with high blood pressure which increases the risk of a stroke *(see box, opposite)*. High-sodium fast foods include hamburgers, sandwiches made with processed meats, and most potato crisps and French fries. In the form of sodium benzoate, a preservative, sodium is also often added to soft drinks. But it is easy to prepare flavourful dishes that are seasoned with little or no salt. Each of the Egg Toast Cups on page 128, for example, has 222 milligrams of sodium, as compared with about 850 milligrams contained in a fried egg sandwich. For lunch or dinner, try Pistou Soup *(page 132)*, which is lower in sodium than most commercial soups because it is made with low-sodium chicken stock and only half a teaspoon of additional salt.

Sugar, too, is pervasive, not only in desserts and snacks, but also in many of the batters that coat fast-food dishes. And commercial soft drinks — other than diet drinks — have an extremely high refined sugar content. Refined sugar has been linked to tooth decay; it also adds extra calories, often in tandem with the fat in rich desserts. You can avoid most of the sugar and fat in desserts by making your own. For example, use a recipe such as Yogurt Fruit Lollies *(page 139)*, which is made with low-fat cottage cheese and yogurt, unsweetened raspberries and only a tablespoon of honey.

If your work or travel schedule makes it difficult for you to prepare nutritious meals, you can still eat less fat, sodium and sugar when dining out. To control fat intake, avoid creamy soups, sauces and dressings; trim all visible fat from meat; and remove the skin from poultry. Instead of a meat sandwich for lunch, try to find a fast-food outlet with a salad bar, where you can get fresh vegetables and fruits, and kidney beans and chick-peas. Resist pickles, mustard, tomato

The Basic Guidelines

For a moderately active adult, Britain's National Advisory Committee on Nutrition Education recommends a diet that is low in fat, high in carbohydrates and moderate in protein. The committee's proposals for the long term suggest that no more than 30 per cent of your calories come from fat, that around 11 per cent come from protein and hence that 55 to 60 per cent come from carbohydrates. A gram of fat equals nine calories, while a gram of protein or carbohydrate equals four calories; therefore, if you eat 2,100 calories a day, you should consume approximately 70 grams of fat, 310 grams of carbohydrate and 60 grams of protein daily. If you follow a low-fat/high-carbohydrate diet, your chance of developing heart disease, cancer and other life-threatening diseases may be considerably reduced.

◆ The nutrition charts that accompany each of the low-fat/high-carbohydrate recipes in this book include the number of calories per serving, the number of grams of fat, carbohydrate and protein in a serving, and the percentage of calories derived from each of these nutrients. In addition, the charts provide the amount of calcium, iron and sodium per serving.

◆ Calcium deficiency may be associated with periodontal diseases — which attack the mouth's bones and tissues, including the gums — in both men and women, and with osteoporosis, or bone shrinking and weakening, in elderly women. The deficiency may also contribute to high blood pressure. The daily allowance for calcium recommended by the United Kingdom Department of Health and Social Security (DHSS) is 500 milligrams a day for men and women. Pregnant and lactating women are advised to consume 1,200 milligrams daily.

◆ Although one way you can reduce your fat intake is to cut your consumption of red meat, you should make sure that you get your necessary iron from other sources. The DHSS suggests a minimum of 10 milligrams of iron per day for men and 12 milligrams for women between the ages of 18 and 54.

◆ High sodium intake is associated with high blood pressure in susceptible people. Most adults should restrict sodium intake to about 2,000 milligrams a day, according to the World Health Organization. One way to keep sodium consumption in check is not to add table salt to food.

sauce and other condiments, which tend to be high in sodium and sugar. And for dessert, instead of ice cream, cake or pie, you can choose fresh fruit with low-fat yogurt.

The best way to ensure that your meals are wholesome is to prepare your own. You can add greater variety to meals and, in addition, save money by taking food from home to work: fast-food meals, like all restaurant meals, are often more expensive than dishes that you can make at home. The following recipes are for foods and beverages that are convenient to take with you and that meet the nutritional guidelines given above. All of them can be prepared ahead of time; many can be frozen if necessary and easily carried in a thermos, an insulated container or even a brown paper bag.

Breakfast

EGG TOAST CUPS

As convenient as a fried egg sandwich, this portable breakfast cuts fat and cholesterol by using only one egg to make two servings.

2 slices fresh, soft wholemeal
   bread
1 large egg
¼ teaspoon dried tarragon
Pinch of salt

Pinch of pepper
45 g (1½ oz) sweet red pepper,
   finely diced
2 tablespoons sliced spring
   onions

Preheat the oven to 190°C (375°F or Mark 5). Fit the bread slices into two small, round, deep moulds each with a 25 cl (8 fl oz) capacity, carefully moulding the bread to conform to the shape. In a small bowl, beat together the egg, tarragon, salt and pepper. Divide the red pepper and spring onions between the bread cups, then pour in the beaten egg and bake for 10 to 12 minutes, or until the egg is set.

Makes 2 servings

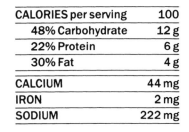

CALORIES per serving	100
48% Carbohydrate	12 g
22% Protein	6 g
30% Fat	4 g
CALCIUM	44 mg
IRON	2 mg
SODIUM	222 mg

Egg Toast Cups

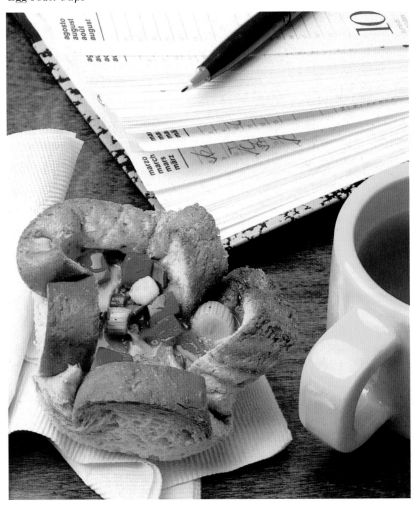

YOGURT WAFFLES

Waffles can be a nutritious convenience dish: store them in the freezer and toast them for breakfast. Boost the calcium content of the waffles by spreading them with yogurt, or top them with fresh berries for added fibre.

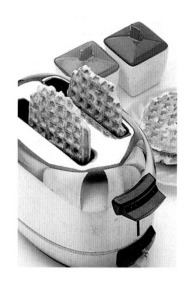

300 g (10 oz) plain flour	**50 cl (16 fl oz) plain low-fat yogurt**
1½ teaspoons baking powder	**2 tablespoons brown sugar**
½ teaspoon bicarbonate of soda	**1 egg, separated, plus 1 egg yolk**
30 g (1 oz) butter or margarine	

Stir together the flour, baking powder and bicarbonate of soda in a large bowl. Melt the butter in a small saucepan over low heat. When the butter is melted, remove the pan from the heat and stir in the yogurt and sugar; set aside. In another large bowl, using an electric mixer, beat the egg white until stiff but not dry; set aside. Lightly beat the egg yolks; add the yolks and the yogurt mixture to the dry ingredients and stir to combine. Stir half of the beaten egg white into the batter, then fold in the remaining egg white.

Grease a waffle iron and preheat it. Using 4 tablespoons of batter for each individual waffle, pour the batter on to the waffle iron and spread it with the back of a spoon (it is thicker than the usual waffle batter). Cook the waffles for about 4 minutes, or according to the waffle-iron manufacturer's instructions, until they are crisp and brown.

Makes about ten 10 cm (4 inch) waffles (5 servings)

CALORIES per serving	330
61% Carbohydrate	50 g
14% Protein	12 g
25% Fat	9 g
CALCIUM	254 mg
IRON	2 mg
SODIUM	338 mg

Note: these waffles actually improve with freezing. Place them in plastic bags, squeeze out as much air as possible and close with a twist-tie. To reheat them, pop them in a toaster, or heat them in a 190°C (375°F or Mark 5) oven for 10 minutes. For an easily transportable breakfast or snack, spread the waffles with strawberry cheese (recipe below).

MUFFINS WITH STRAWBERRY CHEESE

Keep a container of this low-fat, naturally sweet cheese on hand to spread on granary toast or drop scones.

150 g (5 oz) fresh strawberries	**1 tablespoon grated orange rind**
75 g (2½ oz) low-fat cottage cheese	**4 wholemeal muffins**

Wash, dry and hull the strawberries. Place the strawberries, cottage cheese and orange rind in a food processor or blender and process until well blended; the mixture will not be completely smooth. Transfer the mixture to a small bowl, cover and refrigerate for at least 2 hours, or overnight.

Split and toast the muffins. Spread the muffin halves with the strawberry cheese and serve.

Makes 4 servings

CALORIES per serving	155
75% Carbohydrate	31 g
17% Protein	7 g
8% Fat	1 g
CALCIUM	30 mg
IRON	1 mg
SODIUM	304 mg

CALORIES per serving	270
81% Carbohydrate	58 g
12% Protein	8 g
7% Fat	2 g
CALCIUM	241 mg
IRON	1 mg
SODIUM	124 mg

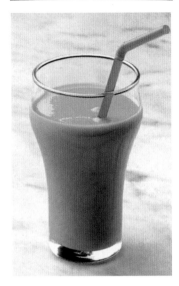

CARROT SHAKE

The vanilla yogurt and banana in this shake hide the carrot flavour, making it taste like a vanilla milk shake. The carrot juice provides more than your daily requirement of vitamin A.

15 cl (¼ pint) carrot juice
12.5 cl (4 fl oz) low-fat vanilla
  yogurt

1 medium-sized banana, peeled
¼ teaspoon pure vanilla extract
1 ice cube

Combine all of the ingredients in a food processor or blender and process until well blended. Pour the shake into a tall glass and serve.   Makes 1 serving

PUMPKIN-SPICE BREAD

For convenience, frozen, individually wrapped portions of this slightly sweet bread can be taken to work or on a journey and eaten after they have thawed.

15 g (½ oz) butter or margarine
12.5 cl (4 fl oz) buttermilk
2 tablespoons honey
2 teaspoons dried yeast
125 g (4 oz) cooked or canned
  pumpkin, mashed

½ teaspoon ground allspice
Pinch of salt
75 g (2½ oz) raisins (optional)
350 g (12 oz) plain flour,
  approximately

Warm the butter and buttermilk in a small saucepan over low heat until the butter melts and the mixture is just tepid. Meanwhile, stir together the honey, yeast and 2 tablespoons of warm water (40-45°C/105-115°F) in a small bowl; set aside for 10 minutes. In a large bowl, stir together the pumpkin, allspice and salt. Stir in the buttermilk and yeast mixtures and the raisins, if using them, then gradually add enough flour to form an elastic dough that pulls away from the sides of the bowl.

Turn the dough out on to a lightly floured board and knead it with floured hands for 5 to 10 minutes, or until the dough is smooth and elastic, kneading in more flour if necessary. Oil a large bowl. Place the dough in the bowl, cover it with a tea towel and let it rise in a draught-free place for 30 to 45 minutes, or until it has doubled in bulk.

Lightly grease a baking sheet. Knock back the dough and shape it into a round loaf. Place the loaf on the baking sheet and leave it to rise again for approximately 30 minutes, or until it has doubled in bulk. Meanwhile, preheat the oven to 190°C (375°F or Mark 5).

With sharp scissors cut a cross in the top of the loaf. Bake the bread for about 35 minutes, or until the loaf sounds hollow when tapped. Transfer the loaf to a rack to cool, then slice the bread and wrap each slice tightly in plastic film for freezing.   Makes 8 servings

CALORIES per serving	210
81% Carbohydrate	43 g
10% Protein	5 g
9% Fat	2 g
CALCIUM	33 mg
IRON	2 mg
SODIUM	50 mg

Lunch

DILLED CRAB SALAD ON A BAGEL

Carry this perishable salad in an insulated container, then cut the bagel and make the sandwich when you are ready to eat it. If you freeze a small can or carton of fruit juice and pack it with the salad, it will keep the food cold all morning and still be well chilled at lunchtime.

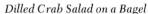

**75 g (2½ oz) fresh or frozen
  crab meat**
2 teaspoons plain low-fat yogurt
1 teaspoon chopped fresh dill
½ teaspoon lemon juice

¼ teaspoon black pepper
30 g (1 oz) thinly sliced cucumber
1 wholemeal bagel
**2 lettuce leaves, torn into bite-
  sized pieces**

Drain the crab meat and remove any bits of shell. Gently stir together the crab meat, yogurt, dill, lemon juice and pepper in a small bowl. Then stir in the cucumber slices; set aside.

Split and toast the bagel. Place the lettuce on one half, spoon the crab salad on to the lettuce and top with the other bagel half. Or divide the lettuce and crab salad between two halves for an open sandwich.   Makes 1 serving

Dilled Crab Salad on a Bagel

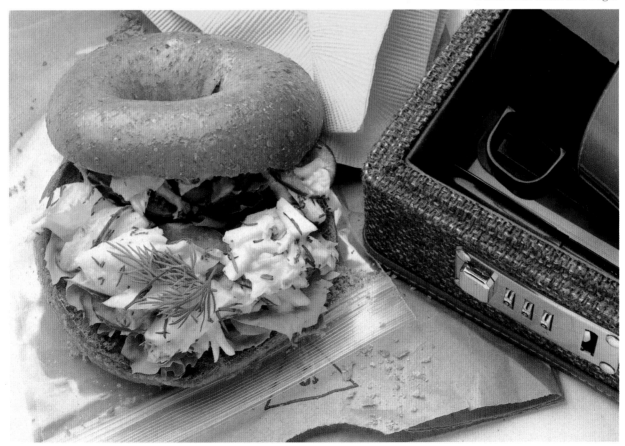

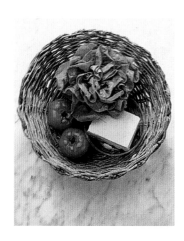

TLT SANDWICH

This version of the BLT (bacon, lettuce, tomato sandwich) replaces high-cholesterol bacon with cholesterol-free tofu, and mayonnaise with yogurt.

300 g (10 oz) firm tofu	**2 tablespoons plain low-fat yogurt**
1 tablespoon tamari	**¼ teaspoon black pepper**
½ teaspoon sugar	**8 slices wholemeal bread**
1 tablespoon prepared	**6 lettuce leaves, shredded**
horseradish	**1 large tomato, thinly sliced**

Drain the tofu, pat it dry and cut it into eight 1 cm (½ inch) thick slices; place them on several thicknesses of paper towels. Place a double layer of paper towels on top, weight with a cutting board and set the tofu aside for about 10 minutes to drain and firm. Meanwhile, line a baking sheet with foil and lightly grease the foil. Stir together the tamari and sugar in a cup; set aside.

Preheat the grill. Arrange the tofu on the baking sheet and sprinkle lightly on both sides with the tamari mixture. Grill the tofu slices 15 cm (6 inches) from the heat for 2 to 3 minutes, or until lightly browned; turn them and grill for another minute. While the tofu is cooking, stir the horseradish, yogurt and pepper together in a small bowl. Toast the bread and spread each slice with the yogurt mixture. Top four slices of toast with lettuce and tomato, divide the tofu among the sandwiches and top with the remaining toast. Makes 4 servings

Note: tamari is a thick, mellow, unrefined soy sauce; look for it in health-food shops and Oriental grocers.

CALORIES per serving	195
52% Carbohydrate	27 g
22% Protein	12 g
26% Fat	6 g
CALCIUM	149 mg
IRON	3 mg
SODIUM	445 mg

PISTOU SOUP

This is a low-fat version of a French soup that traditionally includes large quantities of olive oil and Parmesan.

2 large tomatoes (about 500 g/1 lb),	**75 g (2½ oz) spring onions,**
cored and quartered	**coarsely chopped**
5 garlic cloves, chopped	**25 cl (8 fl oz) low-sodium chicken**
3 tablespoons chopped fresh	**stock**
basil	**175 g (6 oz) cooked red kidney**
2 tablespoons grated Parmesan	**beans**
30 g (1 oz) butter or margarine	**150 g (5 oz) fresh or frozen peas**
1 large potato, peeled and	**1 tablespoon chopped parsley**
coarsely diced (about 200 g/7 oz)	**½ teaspoon salt**
100 g (3½ oz) carrots, sliced	

Put the tomatoes, garlic, basil and Parmesan in a food processor or blender and process just until blended, scraping down the sides of the container with a rubber spatula. Melt the butter in a medium-sized saucepan over medium heat; sauté the potato, carrots and spring onions for 3 to 4 minutes, or until the onions are limp. Add the tomato mixture, stock, kidney beans and 12.5 cl (4 fl oz) of water, and bring to the boil. Cover the pan, reduce the heat to low and simmer for 20 to 25 minutes, or until the potato is tender. Add the peas, parsley and salt, cook for another 5 minutes and serve. Makes 8 servings

CALORIES per serving	120
57% Carbohydrate	17 g
17% Protein	5 g
26% Fat	4 g
CALCIUM	63 mg
IRON	2 mg
SODIUM	210 mg

ITALIAN BREAD SALAD

This Italian-style salad provides more than your daily requirements of vitamins A and C. Pack the vegetables, bread and dressing in a leakproof container in the morning and the salad will be ready to eat at lunchtime.

CALORIES per serving	80
47% Carbohydrate	10 g
16% Protein	3 g
37% Fat	3 g
CALCIUM	33 mg
IRON	2 mg
SODIUM	170 mg

1 sweet red pepper, sliced

1 sweet yellow pepper, sliced

150 g (5 oz) French beans, trimmed

1 small ripe tomato

3 tablespoons vinegar, preferably balsamic

4 tablespoons tomato juice

2 teaspoons walnut oil

¼ teaspoon thyme

Pinch of salt

Pinch of pepper

2½ slices wholemeal bread, cubed (about 60 g/2 oz)

Bring a medium-sized saucepan of water to the boil. Blanch the sweet pepper slices for 3 to 4 minutes, or until barely tender. Reserving the boiling water, remove the blanched peppers with a slotted spoon. Cool the peppers under cold water, drain and set aside. Blanch the beans for about 3 minutes, or until barely tender; cool under cold water, drain and set aside.

For the dressing, core and quarter the tomato, place it in a blender and process until puréed. Add the vinegar, tomato juice, walnut oil, thyme, salt and pepper, and process until blended. Place the blanched vegetables in a large bowl, add the bread cubes and the dressing and toss to combine.

Makes 4 servings

STUFFED CUCUMBER WHEELS

These potassium-rich cucumber rounds contain a low-fat filling. Make them the night before to allow the filling to firm so that they will be ready to take to work in the morning.

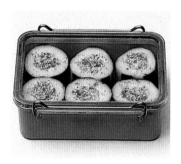

150 g (5 oz) mushrooms, sliced

1 garlic clove, peeled

2 tablespoons chopped onion

1 tablespoon fresh breadcrumbs

1 tablespoon low-fat cottage cheese

1 tablespoon grated Parmesan

2 teaspoons Dijon mustard

¼ teaspoon black pepper

Pinch of salt

Two 25-30 cm (10-12 inch) cucumbers

Pinch of paprika

Place the mushrooms, garlic and 4 tablespoons of water in a small saucepan and bring to the boil over medium heat. Reduce the heat to low, cover and cook for 5 minutes. Drain the mushrooms and garlic and place them in a food processor or blender with the onion, breadcrumbs, cottage cheese, Parmesan, mustard, pepper and salt. Process until puréed and set aside.

Wash the cucumbers. Using a vegetable peeler, remove alternate strips of peel to create a striped effect. Trim the ends and cut each cucumber crosswise into six sections. Using an apple corer or melon baller, remove the seeds. Using a table knife, stuff the cucumber sections with the mushroom mixture, then wrap the sections in plastic film and refrigerate until well chilled. To serve, cut each cucumber section crosswise into two or three pieces and sprinkle with the paprika.

Makes 2 servings

CALORIES per serving	95
62% Carbohydrate	16 g
21% Protein	6 g
17% Fat	2 g
CALCIUM	98 mg
IRON	2 mg
SODIUM	307 mg

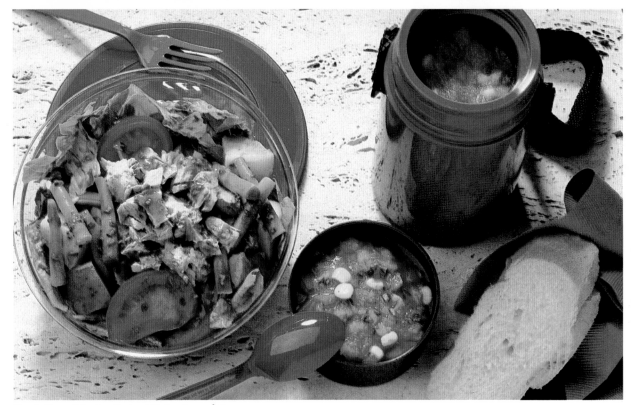

Fresh Tuna Niçoise, Spicy Winter Squash Soup

SPICY WINTER SQUASH SOUP

Most canned soups are very high in sodium, but this soup replaces most of the sodium with spices and adds flavour with vegetables. Freeze portions to eat thawed but still chilled at lunch or keep the soup hot in a thermos.

One 1.25 kg (2½ lb) acorn squash
35 cl (12 fl oz) canned spicy vegetable juice
150 g (5 oz) sweet green pepper, chopped
165 g (5½ oz) fresh or frozen sweetcorn kernels
1 tablespoon chopped fresh basil
Pinch of salt

Preheat the oven to 200°C (400°F or Mark 6). Line a medium-sized baking dish with foil. Halve the squash, remove the seeds and place the squash cut side down in the dish. Bake for 20 to 25 minutes, or until the squash is tender when pierced with a knife. Remove the squash from the oven and allow it to cool for about 15 minutes.

Scoop the squash into a large saucepan and mash it with a potato masher or fork to remove any large lumps (or purée the squash in a food processor or blender). Add 35 cl (12 fl oz) of water, the vegetable juice, green pepper, sweetcorn, basil and salt, and bring to the boil over medium-high heat. Reduce the heat to low and simmer for 10 to 15 minutes. Serve hot, or cool the soup to room temperature and then refrigerate it and serve it chilled.

Makes 6 servings

CALORIES per serving	95
86% Carbohydrate	24 g
9% Protein	3 g
5% Fat	1 g
CALCIUM	60 mg
IRON	2 mg
SODIUM	252 mg

FRESH TUNA NIÇOISE

If you regularly eat tuna with mayonnaise on white bread, this is a low-fat alternative. Unlike mayonnaise, the vinaigrette contains little oil. The vegetables and bread provide complex carbohydrates, while the fish contains high-quality protein.

CALORIES per serving	200
61% Carbohydrate	31 g
20% Protein	10 g
19% Fat	4 g
CALCIUM	44 mg
IRON	2 mg
SODIUM	280 mg

350 g (12 oz) potatoes
150 g (5 oz) French beans, cut into 4 cm (1½ inch) pieces
125 g (4 oz) fresh tuna steak, 2 cm (¾ inch) thick
4 tablespoons red wine vinegar
1 tablespoon virgin olive oil
1 tablespoon Dijon mustard
1 tablespoon chopped fresh chives
Pinch of salt
Pinch of pepper
2 medium-sized tomatoes
250 g (8 oz) cos lettuce, torn into bite-sized pieces
175 g (6 oz) French bread, sliced

Bring a medium-sized saucepan of water to the boil. Scrub the potatoes, place them in the boiling water, cover, reduce the heat to low and simmer for about 20 minutes, or until the potatoes are tender when pierced with a knife. Meanwhile, bring a small saucepan of water to the boil. Blanch the beans for 2 to 3 minutes, cool under cold water and set aside in a colander to drain.

Preheat the oven to 190°C (375°F or Mark 5). Place the tuna in a small baking dish, add 2 tablespoons of water, cover with foil and bake for 10 minutes, or until the fish flakes when tested with a knife. Flake the tuna with a fork, cover loosely and set aside. In a small bowl, whisk together the vinegar, oil, mustard, chives, salt and pepper; transfer half the dressing to a medium-sized bowl. When the potatoes are done, drain them, cool slightly and cut into 2.5 cm (1 inch) cubes. Add them to the larger bowl of dressing and toss to coat. Cut the tomatoes into wedges. Divide the lettuce among six bowls and arrange the potatoes, tomatoes, French beans and tuna on top. Pour the remaining dressing over the salads and serve with the French bread.

Makes 6 servings

DOUBLE POTATO SALAD

Typical delicatessen potato salads are immersed in high-fat dressings. The buttermilk dressing in this recipe is much lower in fat, and the sweet potatoes provide vitamin A.

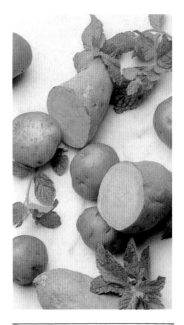

500 g (1 lb) potatoes
500 g (1 lb) orange-fleshed sweet potatoes
5 spring onions
12.5 cl (4 fl oz) buttermilk
12.5 cl (4 fl oz) plain low-fat yogurt
4 tablespoons chopped fresh mint
1 tablespoon brown sugar

CALORIES per serving	170
85% Carbohydrate	37 g
11% Protein	5 g
4% Fat	1 g
CALCIUM	91 mg
IRON	1 mg
SODIUM	50 mg

Scrub the potatoes and sweet potatoes, place them in a large pan and add cold water to cover. Bring to the boil, cover and simmer for about 20 minutes, or until the potatoes are tender when pierced with a knife. (The potatoes may be done a few minutes before the sweet potatoes.) Drain the potatoes and set aside to cool. Meanwhile, coarsely chop the spring onions; set aside. In a large bowl, stir together the buttermilk, yogurt, mint and sugar. When the potatoes are cool, cut them into 2 cm (¾ inch) cubes. Add the potatoes and spring onions to the dressing and toss to combine. Makes 6 servings

GRILLED AUBERGINE AND GARLIC SOUP

CALORIES per serving	55
77% Carbohydrate	11 g
17% Protein	3 g
6% Fat	4 g
CALCIUM	66 mg
IRON	1 mg
SODIUM	52 mg

Aubergine soaks up a lot of oil when it is fried. But this soup is made with grilled aubergine, which is low in fat. The low-sodium chicken stock adds flavour without raising the sodium content.

600 g (1¼ lb) aubergines
1 medium-sized onion
7 garlic cloves
25 cl (8 fl oz) low-sodium chicken stock

1 tablespoon curry powder, or less to taste
Pinch of salt

Preheat the grill. Line a baking sheet with foil. Halve the aubergines and place the halves cut side down on the baking sheet. Place the unpeeled onion and garlic cloves on the baking sheet and grill the vegetables 15 cm (6 inches) from the heat for 20 to 30 minutes, turning the garlic cloves occasionally and removing them if they are done before the aubergine and onion. The onion skin should be dark brown, the garlic amber-coloured and the aubergine almost blackened. Remove the roasted vegetables from the grill and set aside until cool enough to handle.

Scoop the aubergine flesh into a food processor or blender. Peel and add the garlic and onion and process until puréed. Add the stock and curry powder and process until blended. Transfer the purée to a medium-sized saucepan, stir in the salt and 12.5 cl (4 fl oz) of water and bring the soup to the boil over medium-high heat. Reduce the heat to low and simmer the soup for 5 to 7 minutes. Serve hot, or cool the soup to room temperature, refrigerate it for 3 to 4 hours and serve chilled.   Makes 4 servings

BROWN RICE AND VEGETABLE SALAD

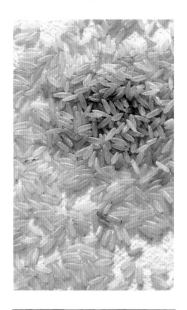

CALORIES per serving	290
74% Carbohydrate	55 g
12% Protein	9 g
14% Fat	5 g
CALCIUM	115 mg
IRON	2 mg
SODIUM	112 mg

A wide-necked thermos flask is ideal for this main-dish salad, which is a good high-fibre alternative to most sandwiches.

750 g (1½ lb) broccoli florets and stems, cut into 1 cm (½ inch) pieces
600 g (1¼ lb) cool, cooked brown rice (250g/8 oz raw)
125 g (4 oz) sweet red pepper, coarsely diced
30 g (1 oz) spring onions, coarsely chopped

2 tablespoons grated Parmesan
2 tablespoons chopped fresh basil
¼ teaspoon black pepper
Pinch of salt
4 tablespoons red wine vinegar
2 teaspoons safflower oil

Bring a large pan of water to the boil. Blanch the broccoli for 1 to 2 minutes; drain and cool under cold water. In a large bowl, combine the cooled broccoli, the rice, red pepper, spring onions, Parmesan, basil, black pepper and salt, and stir to mix. Add the vinegar and oil and toss lightly. Refrigerate the salad for 3 to 4 hours, or until well chilled.   Makes 4 servings

BLACK BEAN AND SWEETCORN CHILI

Even though this chili is meatless, the combination of beans and sweetcorn provides as complete a protein as meat. You can mix up a batch of chili ahead of time and carry it to work in a thermos.

90 g (3 oz) onion, coarsely
   chopped
2 garlic cloves, chopped
1 tablespoon safflower oil
275 g (9 oz) cooked black beans
250 g (8 oz) canned tomatoes,
   with their liquid
1 tablespoon tomato paste

165 g (5½ oz) frozen sweetcorn
   kernels
1 tablespoon chili powder
1 teaspoon ground cumin
1 teaspoon sugar
75 g (2½ oz) sweet green
   pepper, diced

CALORIES per serving	200
63% Carbohydrate	34 g
17% Protein	9 g
20% Fat	5 g
CALCIUM	75 mg
IRON	4 mg
SODIUM	159 mg

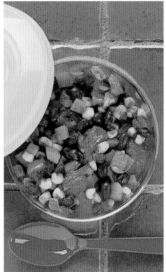

Sauté the onion and garlic in the oil in a medium-sized saucepan over medium heat for 1 to 2 minutes, or until the onion is translucent. Add the beans, tomatoes, tomato paste, sweetcorn, chili powder, cumin and sugar, and stir to combine. Reduce the heat, cover the pan and simmer the mixture for 15 to 20 minutes. Add the green pepper and cook for about 5 minutes more.

Makes 4 servings

CLEMENTINE-ONION SALAD WITH RASPBERRY DRESSING

This combination of fruits, vegetables and cheese provides vitamin C, fibre and some calcium without the fat present in most salad dressings. When packing this meal, keep the dressing and cheese separate; add them only at the last minute.

1 small red onion, thinly sliced
2 clementines or tangerines
30 g (1 oz) fresh raspberries
4 tablespoons raspberry vinegar
2 teaspoons sunflower oil

Pinch of salt
Pinch of pepper
200 g (7 oz) oakleaf lettuce, torn
   into bite-sized pieces
60 g (2 oz) low-fat cottage cheese

Bring a small saucepan of water to the boil. Blanch the onion slices for 30 seconds, or just until limp; drain and pat dry with paper towels. Peel the clementines, removing all the pith; separate the segments and remove and discard the seeds, if any, and the membranes.

In a small bowl, mash the raspberries with a fork. Add the vinegar, oil, salt and pepper, and stir until well blended; set aside. Divide the lettuce among four salad plates and top with the onions and clementines.

Just before serving, sprinkle each salad with 1 tablespoon of cottage cheese and dribble the dressing over the salads.　　　　Makes 4 servings

CALORIES per serving	65
49% Carbohydrate	8 g
16% Protein	3 g
35% Fat	3 g
CALCIUM	36 mg
IRON	1 mg
SODIUM	98 mg

Note: the small, tart clementine is a cross between a Seville orange and a tangerine; unlike a tangerine, it is usually seedless. Raspberry vinegar is a slightly sweetened infusion of the berries in white vinegar. Substitute a mild red wine vinegar if necessary, adding a pinch of sugar if you wish.

Dessert

HERB-GRILLED GRAPEFRUIT

Citrus fruit is one of the best sources of vitamin C. This slightly sweetened dessert tastes good at any temperature, which increases its convenience.

2 medium-sized pink or white grapefruits	**1 tablespoon honey**
	25 to 30 large fresh basil leaves

Preheat the grill. Halve the grapefruits and, using a sharp paring knife, cut between the membranes and the flesh to free the segments. Place the grapefruit halves on a baking sheet and spread about ¾ teaspoon of honey on each half. Place 4 or 5 basil leaves on each half, rubbing the grapefruit with the basil and completely covering the surface of each half with the leaves. Grill the grapefruit 15 cm (6 inches) from the heat for 1 to 2 minutes, or until the honey has melted into the grapefruit and the basil leaves are slightly charred. Discard the charred basil, garnish each grapefruit half with 2 fresh basil leaves and serve hot or at room temperature.   Makes 4 servings

Note: for a different flavour, fresh mint leaves can be substituted for basil.

CALORIES per serving	55
93% Carbohydrate	14 g
5% Protein	1 g
2% Fat	1 g
CALCIUM	23 mg
IRON	Trace
SODIUM	Trace

Herb-Grilled Grapefruit

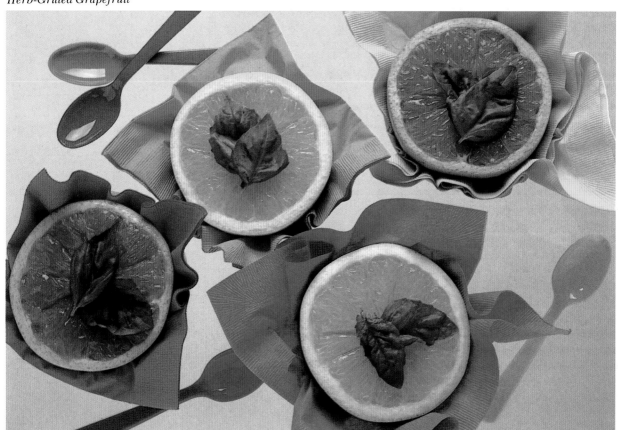

YOGURT FRUIT LOLLIES

About 60 g (2 oz) of ice cream may contain up to 29 grams of mostly saturated fat. Each of these easy-to-carry lollies has just 1 gram of fat.

125 g (4 oz) frozen unsweetened raspberries
2 tablespoons low-fat cottage cheese
1 tablespoon grated lemon rind

1 medium-sized banana, peeled and cut into chunks
1 tablespoon honey
12.5 cl (4 fl oz) plain low-fat yogurt

Place the raspberries, cottage cheese and lemon rind in a blender and process until puréed. Add the banana and honey and process until blended. Transfer the mixture to a small bowl, stir in the yogurt and divide the mixture among four ice-lolly moulds or paper cups. Place the lollies in the freezer for about 2 hours, then insert a wooden stick in the centre of each and freeze for another 6 hours, or until frozen solid. Makes 4 servings

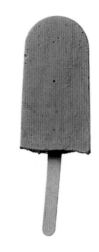

CALORIES per serving	80
78% Carbohydrate	17 g
14% Protein	3 g
8% Fat	1 g
CALCIUM	67 mg
IRON	3 mg
SODIUM	49 mg

CINNAMON BAKED PEARS

Apple-juice concentrate is a versatile natural sweetener. Low-fat fromage frais is a good substitute for cream.

4 firm pears
17.5 cl (6 fl oz) apple-juice concentrate

Grated rind of 1 lemon
½ teaspoon cinnamon
4 tablespoons *fromage frais*

Preheat the oven to 200°C (400°F or Mark 6). Peel, core and halve the pears and place them in a glass baking dish. In a small bowl, combine the apple-juice concentrate, lemon rind and cinnamon; pour the mixture over the pears and bake, uncovered, for 25 to 30 minutes, turning occasionally. Let the pears cool, then cover and refrigate until well chilled. Divide the pears among four dessert plates and top with the *fromage frais*. Makes 4 servings

CALORIES per serving	190
84% Carbohydrate	44 g
3% Protein	1 g
13% Fat	13 g
CALCIUM	32 mg
IRON	1 mg
SODIUM	17 mg

MAPLE PECAN BAKED APPLES

Wrap the apples in foil to take on a winter hike for a high-carbohydrate energy boost that is lower in fat than chocolate bars.

4 medium-sized cooking apples
4 tablespoons pure maple syrup
2 tablespoons finely chopped dried apricots
1 tablespoon grated fresh ginger root

2 tablespoons chopped pecans
1 teaspoon lemon juice
¼ teaspoon grated lemon rind
Pinch of ground cinnamon
4 cinnamon sticks

Preheat the oven to 180°C (350°F or Mark 4). Core the apples, being careful not to cut through the bottoms. In a small bowl, stir together the maple syrup, apricots, ginger, pecans, lemon juice and rind, and ground cinnamon. Divide the filling among the apples and place a cinnamon stick in each apple. Stand the apples in a baking dish and bake for 35 to 40 minutes. Makes 4 servings

CALORIES per serving	180
85% Carbohydrate	42 g
2% Protein	1 g
13% Fat	3 g
CALCIUM	63 mg
IRON	2 mg
SODIUM	3 mg

139

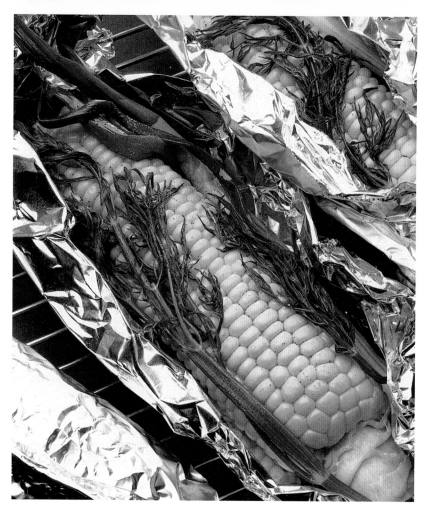

Herbed Sweetcorn

Snacks and Beverages

HERBED SWEETCORN

Flavouring sweetcorn with herbs avoids the fat and sodium that several pats of butter and a heavy sprinkling of salt would add. Cooking vegetables in the oven or on the barbecue conserves more nutrients than boiling.

4 medium-sized ears of sweetcorn	Pinch of salt
15 g (½ oz) butter, melted	4 spring onions
½ teaspoon pepper	8 dill sprigs

Preheat the oven to 190°C (375°F or Mark 5). Husk the sweetcorn, remove the silk and rinse the sweetcorn. Place each cob on a square of foil and brush the sweetcorn lightly with the butter. Season with pepper and salt and place a spring onion and 2 dill sprigs on each cob. Wrap the foil tightly round the sweetcorn and bake for 25 minutes. Serve hot, or refrigerate the sweetcorn in the foil and serve it cold.

Makes 4 servings

CALORIES per serving	110
64% Carbohydrate	20 g
10% Protein	3 g
26% Fat	4 g
CALCIUM	50 mg
IRON	2 mg
SODIUM	71 mg

MELON-BERRY JUICE

Carbonated soft drinks usually contain large amounts of refined sugar, and some contain caffeine. Fruit juices, while not especially low in calories, contain important minerals as well as vitamin C.

2 kg (4 lb) orange-fleshed melon such as cantaloupe or Charentais

125 g (4 oz) fresh raspberries, or frozen unsweetened raspberries, thawed

Halve and seed the melon. Using a spoon or melon baller, scoop out the flesh. If using fresh raspberries, wash them. Place the raspberries in a food processor or blender and process until puréed. Add the melon and continue processing until the fruit is completely liquefied. Serve the juice over ice.

Makes 4 servings

CALORIES per serving	95
85% Carbohydrate	23 g
8% Protein	2 g
7% Fat	1 g
CALCIUM	32 mg
IRON	1 mg
SODIUM	20 mg

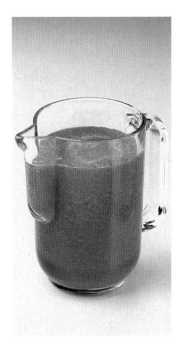

ARTICHOKES WITH GARLIC-ONION DIP

A high-fibre artichoke is just as filling as a high-fat snack such as crisps and the fibre satisfies you without loading on the calories.

2 large globe artichokes
50 cl (16 fl oz) low-sodium chicken stock
1 small onion, peeled
2 garlic cloves, peeled
12 black peppercorns

1 bay leaf
½ teaspoon thyme
Pinch of salt
60 g (2 oz) low-fat cottage cheese
2 teaspoons chopped parsley

Trim the artichoke stems and tough outer leaves. Rinse the artichokes well and place them in a medium-sized saucepan. Add the stock, onion, garlic, peppercorns, bay leaf, thyme, salt and enough water to cover the artichokes. Bring to the boil over medium-high heat, then reduce the heat to low and simmer, covered, for 30 to 40 minutes, or until the bases of the artichokes can be easily pierced with a knife.

Remove the artichokes, onion and garlic from the pan and drain. Place the onion, garlic, cottage cheese and parsley in a blender and process until combined. Serve the artichokes with the garlic-onion dip. Makes 2 servings

CALORIES per serving	120
69% Carbohydrate	23 g
26% Protein	9 g
5% Fat	1 g
CALCIUM	120 mg
IRON	4 mg
SODIUM	318 mg

CINNAMON-PEACHY SHAKE

You can make this shake quickly, and it provides a good supply of calcium, potassium and vitamin A.

1 large peach
12.5 cl (4 fl oz) low-fat vanilla yogurt

1 teaspoon honey
Pinch of cinnamon, or to taste
1 ice cube

Peel, stone and quarter the peach. Place all of the ingredients in a blender and process until well blended. Serve immediately. Makes 1 serving

CALORIES per serving	190
80% Carbohydrate	40 g
13% Protein	7 g
7% Fat	2 g
CALCIUM	204 mg
IRON	Trace
SODIUM	75 mg

ACKNOWLEDGEMENTS

The editors wish to thank Norma MacMillan and
Christine Noble.

Index prepared by Ian Tucker.